Pesticides and Global Health

Anthropology and Global Public Health:
Critical Approaches and Constructive Solutions

This series publishes books at the intersection of medical anthropology and global public health that use robust theoretical and ethnographic insights to develop practical public health solutions. Using accessible language to communicate complex global health problems, they examine concrete failures and successes in global health through an anthropological lens emphasizing historical, ecological, political, and sociocultural contexts. They also showcase leading methodological approaches, both qualitative and quantitative. The series publishes books in two formats: Tightly orchestrated edited volumes consisting of original writing by leading scholars advance major themes and methods and provide instructors with important new tools for integrating medical anthropology and global public health into the curricula of both disciplines. Short, single-authored books focused on a particular global health problem are constructed in three sections: a broad introduction to the problem and literature to date; a case study illustrating key issues and methods; and constructive solutions, including broader implications for application in public health programs.

ANTHROPOLOGY AND GLOBAL PUBLIC HEALTH

Pesticides and Global Health

Understanding Agrochemical Dependence and Investing in Sustainable Solutions

Courtney Marie Dowdall and Ryan J. Klotz

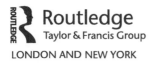

Routledge
Taylor & Francis Group

LONDON AND NEW YORK

First published 2014 by Left Coast Press, Inc.

Published 2016 by Routledge
2 Park Square, Milton Park, Abingdon, Oxon OX14 4RN
711 Third Avenue, New York, NY 10017, USA

Routledge is an imprint of the Taylor & Francis Group, an informa business

Library of Congress Cataloging-in-Publication Data
Dowdall, Courtney.
    Pesticides and global health : understanding agrochemical dependence and investing in sustainable solutions / Courtney Dowdall and Ryan J. Klotz.
    pages cm. — (Anthropology and global public health ; Volume 1)
    Summary: "This concise, accessible introduction to understanding agricultural chemicals and public health combines a broad synthesis on a global scale with rich ethnographic narratives on a human scale. Drawing on epidemiology, policy analysis, and social science research on the global commodity chain, the authors describe the system of global agrochemical dependence that constitutes a major threat to human health. Then they draw readers into the lush mountainsides of highland Guatemala, telling personal stories of farmers, their experiences with public health programs, their struggles against agrichemical dependence, and their innovations in sustainable agriculture. Finally, they show how this kind of qualitative, multi-level analysis holds practical lessons for public health. This engaging, brief text is an ideal supplement for courses in global health, introducing students to key concepts with broad coverage and engrossing ethnographic detail"— Provided by publisher.
    Includes bibliographical references and index.
    ISBN 978-1-61132-304-7 (hardback) — ISBN 978-1-61132-305-4 (paperback) — ISBN 978-1-61132-702-1 (consumer ebook)
    1. World health.   2. Agricultural chemicals—Environmental aspects.   I. Klotz, Ryan J.
II. Title.
    RA441.D69 2014
    363.17'92—dc23
                    2013029132

ISBN 978-1-61132-304-7 hardback
ISBN 978-1-61132-305-4 paperback

Cover design by Piper Wallis
Text design by Detta Penna

Contents

Preface

Guatemala has been the recipient of an endless parade of international aid and development organizations. Chicken coops, community gardens, weaving cooperatives, internet cafes, microenterprises—the list of projects brought to the Guatemalan people is exhaustive. Our research in Guatemala began in 2007 as an investigation of a recycling plant constructed several years earlier and intended to clean up one of the country's most agriculturally productive and chemically polluted hamlets. A Norwegian development agency had donated funds to build a facility and purchase trucks that would collect compostable waste from the nearby market and convert this organic matter into chemical-free fertilizer. Everyone we had questioned about the recycling plant had confidently affirmed that the facility was a success, functioning as planned. One resident explained how they routinely purchased fertilizer from the plant. No one offered so much as a hint of doubt regarding the status of the plant.

From the roadside bus stop a few miles away, the plant appeared to be open for business and filled to the brim with materials waiting to be recycled. It was not until we could make out the details of the collected objects that we realized the plant had been converted into a rat-infested trash dump, vultures circling overhead, swarms of flies blooming underfoot with each step toward the facility. Unfortunately, like so many other well-intended development efforts, the infrastructure and customs of this village were not prepared to support the long-term success of the recycling plant.

Why would so many repeat the official story of the plant's success, even overcompensating with their own anecdotes? News in a small town travels quickly. It was inconceivable that the fate of the recycling plant had not reached a single soul in our investigation. After our initial disappointment with the "failed" project had subsided, we realized what a valuable lesson we had learned in the process.

What this ill-fated research project led us to understand was that the residents of Guatemala, of this hamlet in particular, knew there was a problem with their agricultural system. Beyond the recycling plant, they had received so many trainings and donations intended to help them curb their chemical usage, clean up their rivers, and properly dispose of their waste, that the message had been ingrained in their moral compass. Despite all the support they had received, however, and all their honest intentions to adopt these best practices, they still felt incapable of making the recommended changes. Rather than focus solely on the ruination of the recycling plant, we shifted our attention to projects and workshops that were ongoing to better understand why some development inter-ventions were deemed useful and incorporated into agricultural practices while others were perceived as unreasonable and subsequently abandoned.

In subsequent summers, and during an eighteen-month stay be-tween 2009 and 2010, we conducted interviews and surveys, packaged vegetables, picked coffee, toured markets, attended meetings, visited fields, sorted beans, and chatted with purchasers of agricultural products. We hiked, bussed, shuttled, and caught pickups to the remote mountaintop and volcano-side villages where we worked. We shared three meals a day and innumerable tortillas with families in the countryside. We shared cof-fee, chocolate, beers, and bread with our progressive friends in the city. We talked about school, families, illness, civil war, holiday plans, soccer games, trade agreements, and presidential elections. We basked in the occasional compliment for our Spanish language skills and learned to nimbly deflect the frequent jokes about being thirty-something and childless.

As a married couple and a research team, we were fortunate to have access to both women at home alone and men at work in fields. We had the benefit of two pairs of ears, two sets of eyes, and a constant source of moral support. When one of us felt discouraged, the other summoned the optimism to persevere. If one of us missed an opportunity to pursue a pithy interview topic, the other was poised to interject. Where one strug-gled to phrase a question just so and elicit the information we needed, the other was at the ready with an alternative. Our dispositions are just as complementary in the field as they are in writing, and we hope this translates into a strength of this book.

After spending so much time in so many heartfelt discussions of the future of Guatemala's food systems, communities, and families, we concerned ourselves with sharing what we have learned with as broad an audience as possible. Perhaps the biggest lesson we took away from work was that, though Guatemala has been the recipient of an outpouring of international aid, and much more aid is needed as the country struggles to recover from the civil violence of the 1980s and 1990s, the form and function of development support must be more focused, constructive, and collaborative. The obstacles preventing the most well-intended international development efforts from taking root and effecting positive change in Guatemala are multifaceted and comprise both internal and external factors. But we hope that our analysis of global processes and the ways they affect the lives of individuals and their families will enhance efforts to promote the kind of broad structural change that addresses the specific concerns of the spectrum of stakeholders involved in agriculture in Guatemala and many other exporting nations. By designing public health intervention strategies such as safe pesticide use and ecological production campaigns that address big-picture concerns as well as grassroots perspectives, we believe that individuals in all stages of agricultural production can be part of the solution to the multifaceted problem of agrochemical use around the world.

Acknowledgments

We would like to thank the many friends, families, colleagues, and professors whose support and collaboration have made this work possible.

In the field, residents of the communities in which we worked opened the doors to their homes, invited us to sit at their dinner tables, and generously shared their thoughts and experiences. The organizations that facilitated our work served as a sounding board for ideas and offered the feedback we needed to create a more revelatory study. Our friends at Celas Maya and Al Natur patiently helped us cultivate the conversational skills and cultural understanding that helped us conduct fieldwork more graciously.

We appreciate the efforts of Liliana Goldín and Guillermo Grenier for their mentorship during the entirety of our graduate careers and for their involvement in these projects, from the preliminary stages to completion.

We would like to acknowledge Florida International University, the National Science Foundation, the United States Department of Agriculture, and the Tinker Foundation for financial support that made this work possible.

Finally, we would like to thank our families for their love and patience throughout the entire research process. They could never understand just how vital all the long-distance phone calls, letters of encouragement, and constant reassurances were to seeing this endeavor through to the end.

Introduction

From high altitude vegetable growing regions to lower altitude areas of coffee production, the most striking feature of a drive through Guatemala is how green everything is. After the first harrowing moments in a chicken bus, amazement at the sheer volume of passengers crammed into a single vehicle, and the fear of the ever wider and faster cliffside turns, a traveler finally surrenders to the breathtaking view of the Guatemalan countryside. As the bus climbs the mountains into the Western Highlands region, women pull sweaters around their shoulders and mothers bundle their babies tightly in blankets rigged up like a sling. The heat from fellow passengers provides a welcome block against the cool air as the bus passes through the misty vegetable growing countryside. Swathes of squares cut into the hills rise and fall in soft mounds, with borders demarcating plots of onion, potato, lettuce, cabbage, and carrot.

As the bus reaches the city of Quetzaltenango, passengers scramble to collect their belongings from the luggage racks overhead. Women grab baskets and boxes and cord-wrapped bundles, adroitly placing them atop their heads as they descend to the street, never faltering, never second-guessing a single step. They carry their goods to the various markets of Xela—Democracia, Terminal, Parque Central, Las Flores—where they set up for the day. Dressed in *traje* (traditional attire), they sit on the ground with their vegetables displayed in baskets before them and their scales set beside them, each one offering the same selection of radish, carrot, and onion as the next. After selling everything they brought, they bring home the goods they purchased with their earnings—sugar, rice, beans, eggs, oil.

As the traveler switches buses and continues further west, the air becomes heavy and damp as moisture beads up on the foreheads of passengers, who nod to sleep with the swaying of the bus in the tropical heat. Those still awake fight with the windows in hopes of letting in a stream of fresh air. The patchwork hillsides give way to temperate rainforest, where dense mountainsides rise in a lush, vibrant wall on one side of the bus

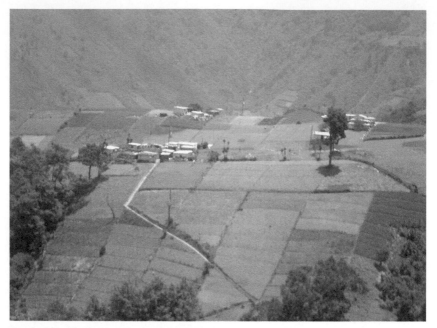

Figure I.1.   Patchwork agricultural fields.

and drop to a ravine on the other, with specks of color from wildflowers like the pink *quinceañera* running rampant throughout the woods. As the bus reaches the market in Retalhuleu Terminal, passengers anxiously peel their sticky legs from the vinyl of the bench seats and eagerly hand over a few bills to the first vendor to pass by with a bucket of sodas on ice.

In contrast to the green and expansive agricultural zones of rural Guatemala, the markets are tight and crowded with every ware imaginable, from foods to cleaning solutions to plastic chairs to baby chicks. Men hauling cartloads of bananas and oranges offer cut slices from their fruits and race one another to sell them by the dozen. Dry goods vendors surround themselves with three-foot tall bags of chilies, spices, and coffee beans, reluctantly storing at the end of the day whatever remains in the burlap sack.

Though the agriculturalists of Guatemala dutifully trek to the market each day to earn their income, they relish their return to the countryside. Ask any farmer how she feels about life in the city and she will not hesitate to tell you that there is no contest: "In the city you have to pay for everything, while in *el campo* (the countryside) we have everything. In *el campo*, you have your own land, where you can grow whatever you need."

But despite this popular image, life in rural Guatemala is increasingly higher maintenance than memory fondly suggests. With all the

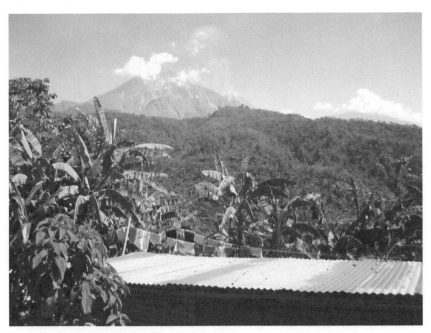

Figure I.2.   Volcano-Oside coffee plantation.

conveniences and improvements of modernizing society—electrical lines linking rooftops in even the remotest villages, high school–level education in nearby cities, bus service to transport students, and cell phone reception on the steep slopes of the Santa Maria Volcano—come increased costs of living. At the same time, globalizing society has expanded the opportunities for Guatemalans to earn money; they now grow new varieties of vegetables and sell coffee to an array of markets. The relative simplicity of life in rural Guatemala is a more bucolic image than the complicated reality of contemporary livelihoods.

Agriculture is of particular economic importance in the developing world. Among developing countries worldwide, 60 percent of the population is employed primarily in agriculture (Hogstedt et al. 2007). In Latin America alone, 112 million people are supported by agricultural work. In Central America in particular, the livelihood of 50 percent of the population depends on farming activities (London et al. 2002). For the billions of people across the world who incorporate agriculture into their livelihood strategies, the global market presents a conundrum of opportunities and difficult choices. Specifically, the introduction of chemical inputs into agriculture has allowed farmers to increase their outputs, grow unfamiliar vegetables in inhospitable regions, and manipulate the quality of their produce to fit preferences of international markets. But the free flow of

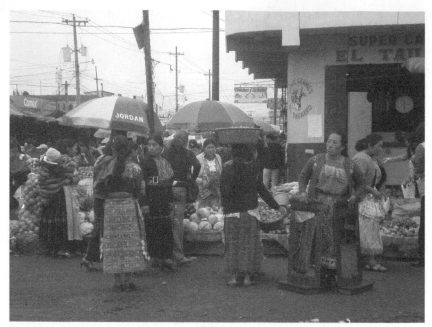

Figure I.3.   Market offerings in Quetzaltenango.

products is a double-edged sword that brings opportunities to farmers in remote places, increasing the number of actors in the global market and raising the bar to be a competitive player. In order to play the game, farmers see little choice but to go all-in with the most powerful and effective chemical inputs they can afford.

Researchers have long described the inertia of this cycle of increasing production, intensifying competition, and then augmenting chemical application to further increase production as the "product price" treadmill. As a result, farmers' profits are eroded by the constantly rising costs of adopting new agricultural technology (Cochrane 1958). This treadmill continues in modern agriculture, and presents a particular foil to efforts in developing nations that have banked their economic growth on agricultural expansion. In Guatemala, the product price treadmill continues to affect farmers as they are forced to spend increasing amounts on inputs such as fertilizers and pesticides just to match the production of their neighbors, watching in frustration as their meager earnings slip through their fingers.

Beyond the economic costs of agrochemical use, pesticides, herbicides, and fertilizers present a number of additional costs to global public health; namely, the burns, headaches, gastrointestinal distress, and respiratory illnesses that result from exposure to and misuse of hazardous

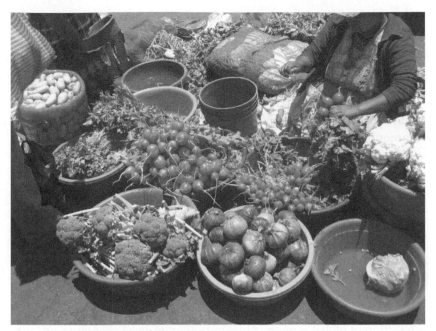

Figure I.4.   Market offerings in Quetzaltenango.

agrochemicals. Making matters worse, though the global economy has increased farmers' access to the chemicals they rely on to remain competitive, globalization generally has not delivered the resources that mitigate the dangers of agrochemical use—education, health care, and the socioeconomic status to advocate for their own safety. The chronic headaches, rashes, and gastritis that are facts of life in rural Guatemala are often attributable to chemical exposure, though the general poor health of farmers can mask the source of these ailments.

Despite warnings, educational campaigns, and regulations, the accounts of agrochemical poisoning are still mounting, leaving researchers and governing bodies to wonder at the shortcomings of their solutions. The international community—in the form of the United Nations World Health Organization (WHO), Environment Programme (UNEP), and Food and Agriculture Organization (FAO)—has made a number of efforts to regulate the flow of the most dangerous agrochemicals and train farmers in best practices for chemical application. However, the worst offenders persist in making their way into the hands of susceptible farmers, who continue to endanger themselves, their families, and their communities in the name of economic survival.

Why does agrochemical use and misuse persist in the face of health and environmental dangers? This book offers an ethnographic perspective of this problem that paints a more holistic picture of the reasons why farmers continue to rely on agrochemicals and, subsequently, offers more enlightened solutions to the quagmire of agrochemical dependence. In the first chapter, we tell the story of how agrochemicals were introduced to the developing world as a means to accelerate economic development and meet the needs of global markets. We discuss various health threats posed by the more nefarious agrochemicals. Focusing on the products commonly used in Guatemala, we review epidemiological studies of agrochemicals as a threat to public health and the reasons why there remains a lack of consensus concerning the causal links between these chemicals and specific health threats. We conclude with a brief history of international regulations that have attempted to halt or restrict the flow of these products in the global market.

In the second chapter, we examine agrochemical use as a threat to global public health, as the risks and dangers are amplified in the precarious health environments that farmers in the developing world so often inhabit. In exploring the complex political, cultural, and economic reasons why these products continue to be used and abused, we look at the interaction of global economic integration, state-level economic austerity policies, armed conflict, and disenfranchisement of rural populations that leaves farmers in developing countries such as Guatemala particularly vulnerable to the hazards of agrochemical use.

In the third and fourth chapters, we provide ethnographic case studies from two major industries in Guatemala—coffee and vegetable cultivation—to illustrate the myriad pressures that push farmers to continue use of dangerous agrochemicals despite their knowledge of the long- and short-term dangers of these products. Through the stories of small coffee growers and vegetable farmers, we highlight a number of socioeconomic treadmills that belie agrochemical use in rural Guatemala. Ultimately, we identify urgent economic needs, overwhelming strains on household labor, and a dearth of information on proper chemical use or alternative techniques—all exacerbated by a fragile infrastructure—as drivers of risky agrochemical use. In the end, however, these cases offer examples of farmers who are escaping the momentum of these socioeconomic treadmills to strike a balance between maintaining a household in the present and securing a livelihood for the future.

Over the course of our four years of research in vegetable and coffee growing communities in Guatemala, farmers shared tragic stories: heartbreaking moments of complete economic ruin precipitated by the need to care for an ill family member, total devastation at hectares of cabbages destroyed by the infamous whitefly, women abandoned by husbands who sought their fortunes in the United States. But they also shared their stories of triumph: a widow who earned enough in agriculture to give her children the educational opportunities she never had, a timid young man who grew into a position of leadership after volunteering to take charge of a coffee processing facility, a community elder who now imparts to his grandchildren the wisdom of organic techniques that had so long been trumped by high-tech chemical expertise and have only recently regained esteem. Though the painful stories are essential to understanding the gravity of the agrochemical problem in the developing world, our attention was instead drawn to the hope and optimism that exists among many farmers.

By sharing the accounts of these victories, some small and some quite significant, we aim to communicate both the valiant efforts made by farmers to protect their families and the high stakes of experimenting with new agricultural practices. We hope that the cases related in this book will contribute new perspectives on the lingering health threats of hazardous chemicals, illustrating the complexity of concerns underlying farmers' persistent use of them. We add to the growing body of literature addressing rural livelihood strategies by outlining the many factors that farmers must take into consideration when determining how to invest their scarce resources. This book also demonstrates the value of anthropological research to conceptualizing global health threats and designing more effective, comprehensive, and innovative solutions to such multifaceted problems as toxic chemical use in agricultural production. Ultimately, we hope that the success stories we describe here convey the faith and optimism among farmers in Guatemala that there is an alternative to agrochemical reliance and the benefits of their efforts have yet to be realized to a full extent.

The experiences of Guatemalan farmers offer positive reinforcement for the innovative solutions already being implemented by international aid, public health, and development programs, and help to highlight further opportunities to combat the complex problem of hazardous agrochemical use. We intend to demonstrate the great risks being taken and the sacrifices being made by farmers seeking an end to the cycle of running to stand still. These stories provide proof that there *are* avenues to escape the many overlapping treadmills that fuel the chemical production cycle. Many of these routes just have yet to be mapped.

Chapter 1

Global Agricultural Markets
and Standardization

Over the past several decades, the production and circulation of agricultural goods has undergone a process of heightening integration on a global scale. From the planting and cultivation of export crops by farmers around the world, to the placement of farm products on the shelves of major supermarkets across the United States and other developed nations, global agriculture is a mammoth industry that employs over 22 percent of the world's population (Smith et al. 2008: 167). In recent years, the agricultural sector has progressively come under the tight control of a few multinational actors. More and more, each step in the chain from farm to table must be managed in the interest of meeting the needs of global markets.

This chapter focuses on how the pressures of the global market condition the activities of large-scale distributors of agricultural goods. The need for profitability in the coffee and vegetable trades gives rise to specific forms of organization, standards for quality, and relations of power in their respective distribution chains. These forms of trade structure the ways in which agricultural production changes to meet industrial needs. This chapter demonstrates how large-scale actors like coffee roasters and supermarket chains struggle to secure predictability, standardization, and the minimization of risks in agriculture—an activity that is inherently unpredictable and risky.

Efforts to standardize agrarian commodity production have contributed to the rise of a multibillion dollar industry (Buccini 2004: 8) that attempts to realize this goal by modernizing agriculture through technology and chemical-based farming. During the post-war era of the 1940s and 1950s, agrochemical pesticides, high-yielding hybrid seeds, and other agro-technologies were widely seen as the solution to the problems of agricultural production and even world hunger. Consequently, an agrochemical industry has developed, primarily in the United States and Europe, to supply growing global demand. The use and circulation of pesticides has seen staggering jumps since the mid-twentieth century.

19

According to some estimates, sales of registered pesticides doubled every ten years between 1945 and 1985 (WHO/UNEP 1990 cited in Dich et al. 1997: 422). By the early 1990s, over two million metric tons of chemical pesticides were sold worldwide with a total value of nearly 26 billion dollars (Dich et al. 1997: 423). Despite some signs of diminished growth, pesticide sales continued in much the same fashion throughout the early 2000s. Approximately 1.7 billion pounds of pesticides were exported from U.S. ports alone between 2001 and 2003 (Smith et al. 2008: 167). Total global exports, however, are much higher, as this figure does not include agrochemicals shipped from other major exporters, including Germany and Switzerland. Overall, current use of pesticides totals about 2.3 million tons dispersed annually around the world (Harris and McCartor 2011: 27); total sales of pesticides have grown from 30 billion dollars in 1999 to over 40 billion in 2008 (Pesticide Action Network (PAN) 2010: 3). According to World Bank estimates, global production of agrochemicals is expected to exceed 1995 production levels by approximately 85 percent by 2020, with greater proportions of chemicals being produced by, and exported to, the developing world (Buccini 2004: 10).

In recent years, many agrochemicals have come under increasing scrutiny for their observed and potential effects on human and environmental health. The risks have not escaped the attention of international organizations and regulators. In light of mounting evidence linking human exposure to certain agrochemicals with the prevalence of cancer, respiratory illnesses, neurological disease, and other health risks, institutions such as the WHO and the FAO have developed several key international agreements to stem or severely restrict the spread of these chemical compounds (see Buccini 2004).

Despite the best efforts of these organizations and widespread acceptance of international bans and participation in regulatory agreements, however, the health and environmental threats posed by the global circulation of agrochemicals persist. According to WHO estimates, over 3 million cases of acute pesticide poisoning occur annually, while long-term exposure to pesticides is thought to be responsible for more than 700,000 cases of chronic illness per year (PAN 2010: 6). The vast majority of these cases are concentrated among populations in the developing world.

In this chapter, we argue that agrochemicals remain a prime threat to the health and environmental well-being of farmers in the developing world because of a set of interrelated processes occurring at the international, national, and local levels. Cochrane's agricultural treadmill does much to explain why farmers and their families continue to be exposed to toxic agrochemicals. However, to develop a full understanding of the persistence of the agrochemical threat, the treadmill concept must be applied more broadly to numerous sociocultural and economic processes that condition farmer decisions concerning agrochemical use, a topic explored in later chapters.

The forces driving global agricultural chains

Agriculture has become a global activity. Recent advances in telecommunication and transportation technologies make it possible for consumers to go into most supermarkets around the world and choose from a variety of farm products that have recently arrived from any given country. Supermarket chains and big-box stores in Canada, the United States, Europe, or Japan are able to arrange large purchases of agricultural goods, issue packaging specifications for their products, pay for express shipping, and receive their products in less than twenty-four hours. Along with these advances in export and communication technologies, a demand for coordination across borders and strategic management of complex agricultural systems has arisen to meet the requirements of globally competitive businesses.

The need for tight integration of every step in the process, from the planting of seeds to the sales of foods to final consumers, has led numerous observers of agricultural commodities to refer to these interlocking stages of production and distribution as "global value chains" (Bair 2005, Gereffi et al. 2005, Kaplinsky 2004). Using this metaphor, researchers show how different forms of organization and transactions take shape at each "link" in a product's chain. Research on global value chains has demonstrated how the requirements for circulating different commodities give rise to distinct sets of relationships between actors and the systems by which products, profits, and power are distributed. Further, global value chain research has also shown how the logistical needs of global circulation require specific kinds of organization and divisions of tasks. These organizational strategies must be adequately efficient and routinized to function in an increasingly competitive world market for agricultural goods (Dolan and Humphrey 2000).

Agricultural value chains are distinct from those of numerous other commodities because they are "buyer-driven" systems (Kaplinsky 2004, Ponte 2002, Dolan and Humphrey 2000). They diverge from "producer-driven" chains for specialized goods, in which producers have a fair amount of power because they possess machinery and expertise that is not easily copied. By contrast, agricultural chains are dominated by large buyers whose power has been fortified by recent consolidations in the industry for agricultural goods.

In both coffee (Ponte 2002, Pendergrast 1999) and fresh vegetable (Konefal et al. 2007, Dolan and Humphrey 2000) circulation chains, the past two decades have been characterized by a rapid cornering of the industries by a handful of multinational firms operating in the global north. At the same time, the number of suppliers—exporters and farmers—has remained constant or increased. As a result, while producers were once able to choose the best terms of trade among a variety of interested purchasers, they now sell the majority of their produce to only one or two large-scale supermarket chains or coffee roasters. For this reason, it is far easier for these "lead firm" (Gereffi 1994) purchasers to switch suppliers of a product than it is for suppliers to find new purchasers (Dolan and Humphrey 2000). In effect, this situation creates a power imbalance wherein large buyers have the freedom to manipulate the other links in the chain to suit their own needs for capital accumulation. These buyers' specifications for product quality, volume, and supply "drive" the modes of production and shape the distribution of agricultural products by other stakeholders in their respective chains. Suppliers are left with the choice either to conform to such specifications or to risk losing out on a contract with an increasingly short list of purchasers.

Quality and production standards of supermarket chains

Although large supermarket chains, coffee roasters, and other purchasers of global agricultural goods are able to harness a great deal of power in their dealings with farmers, exporters, and other suppliers, they continue to struggle with a special set of challenges and barriers to generating a profit. Overall, large-scale buyers of agricultural commodities must minimize unpredictability in their products and supply chains. This drive is in constant tension with the fundamental natural forces upon which agricultural production is based. Agriculture is inherently tied to changes in the weather and a host of highly varied social and environmental circumstances in the producing countries where cultivation takes place. The development of a hurricane that destroys a coffee crop in a Central American nation, for example, can lead to shortages and price spikes for the crop in the global market. Changes in growing conditions can affect product quality or supply, introducing an element of uncertainty that must be mitigated in the interests of securing a successful value chain and business model.

Because the success of retailers like supermarkets and coffee roasters depends heavily on their reputation among their consumers, sourced produce that fails to meet prevailing standards for quality in agricultural markets can create a number of problems. In order to remain competitive, it is essential that retailers ensure a normal and predictable supply of products in sufficient volumes that meet the quality expectations of markets and consumers around the world. The inability to provide products of a consistent quality can be devastating for farmers, especially in the increasingly competitive global markets where a few retailers compete for a fixed consumer base (Dolan and Humphrey 2000, Pendergrast 1999). Establishing and maintaining the reputation of their brands in terms of quality is essential to retailer success. For this reason, supermarkets or coffee roasters seek to keep consumers from switching to a competitor's product by offering agricultural goods that are consistent in supply, appearance, taste, and other markers of quality. As a result, most lead firms in buyer-driven value chains such as those for coffee and vegetables maintain specific minimum standards to which the goods they purchase must conform. This system of passing product quality and production standards down the entire value chain, called "value-chain governance," places the burden of assuring quality on exporters and farmers, who now bear the risk of growing a product that purchasers may be unwilling to buy at harvest time (Jaffee 2007, Fischer and Benson 2006, Mutersbaugh 2002).

In sum, lead-firm retailers attempt to minimize risks to the profitability of their ventures through value chain governance and the development and enforcement of minimum standards for agricultural goods. These mechanisms constitute an effort on the part of retailers to develop an edge over competitors by sourcing a steady and predictable supply of products of an acceptable quality. However, try as they might, maintaining rigid quality standards is a complicated task for farmers of coffee and fresh vegetables, as we will demonstrate in the following sections. Beyond these basic generalizations of global agricultural chains, stakeholders in the fresh vegetables and coffee industries face distinct sets of challenges that nevertheless result in similar approaches to securing the right conditions for profitability and capital accumulation. A brief breakdown of each of these chains illustrates the specific processes and barriers confronted by purchasers and how the use of modern agricultural technologies, specifically agrochemicals, becomes the solution. Though the value chains in which coffee and vegetable farmers participate vary in several key ways, the need to continue supplying produce according to the rigid specifications of retailers can lead farmers of both products to practice similar farming strategies that have the potential to pose serious threats to public health.

Aesthetic standards of consumers

Even among the largest supermarket retailers competition remains fierce. The biggest companies often secure their market shares at the expense of smaller players. For example, in the United States in the early 1980s, the top five national supermarkets controlled just over a quarter of the total countrywide supermarket sales in fresh produce. This figure changed dramatically by 2004, with the top five controlling more than 48 percent of all sales (McTaggart and Heller 2005: 50, cited in Konefal et al. 2007). With the elimination of many small and specialty food retailers from the market, large chains now engage in heated competition for smaller pieces of the consumer market. According to observers (Konefal et al. 2007, Dolan and Humphrey 2000), the rapid consolidation of the fresh fruit and vegetable trade has had far-reaching impacts for the industry in terms of competition, supply procurement, and value chain governance.

The rules of competition in fresh vegetables now center on consumer demands in terms of eye appeal, year-round availability, and uniformity. For this reason, supermarkets have developed specific aims for their sourcing activities, standards for produce, and overall governance of their value chains. In order to ensure a reliable stream of farm produce from exporting countries, supermarket chains contract with a few large exporters who are responsible for aggregating the contracted amount of produce from local farms. In both European (Dolan and Humphrey 2000) and North American (Fischer and Benson 2006) supply chains, supermarket buyers hold these intermediary firms responsible for enforcing standards to ensure that contracted produce meets quality and safety qualifications before hitting the grocers' shelves.

With varying degrees of involvement on the part of their northern purchasers, exporters have become increasingly involved in changing the production process of their supplying farmers to meet these quality standards. To maintain positive working relationships with sourcing retailers, local suppliers and exporters strive to secure sufficient volumes of large, uniform, blemish-free produce that is free from evidence of disease or chemical contamination. Critically, they transfer the responsibility and cost of meeting these supermarket standards to farmers by inserting them directly into contracts with contracted farmers (Fischer and Benson 2006), making on-site visits to the fields of contracted farmers (Conroy et al. 1996), and conducting inspections of submitted produce. Any violations of the standards for product quality or production can lead to outright rejection of a farmer's entire harvest.

This arrangement clearly places a large part of the burden of ensuring product quality on the shoulders of farmers. According to many of the farmers we encountered in our research, purchasers do in fact routinely reject contracted produce that does not conform to specific quality standards. In the mid-1990s in Guatemala, for example, farmers reported that at least 25 percent of their produce was rejected at the packaging shed for failure to meet contracted standards (Conroy et al. 1996). More recent data show Guatemalan exporters reject approximately 15 percent of all broccoli harvests submitted by farmers based on appearance alone (Fischer and Benson 2006: 29).

Competition between individual farmers to meet standards for quality and volume in the fresh produce value chain parallels the competition among large supermarket chains. Farmers desperate to sell a perishable crop like fresh snow peas will do whatever it takes to ensure that their harvests meet contract specifications concerning quantity, volume, and cosmetic, sanitary, and chemical standards. If they fail to meet these specifications or attempt to work outside contractual agreements with large suppliers, farmers are left to fend for themselves in the local open markets, where prices are wildly unpredictable and subject to even greater competitive pressures.

Supply standards of international commodity brokers

Coffee has a much longer history as a global commodity than do fresh vegetables. However, the contemporary coffee market transformed considerably following the fall of the International Coffee Agreement (ICA) in 1989 (Bacon 2005, Taylor 2005, Ponte 2002). Forged in the early 1960s at a UN Coffee Conference in New York, the ICA aimed to create a stable coffee price for exporting farmers and producing countries. This agreement between buying and producing nations attempted to set stable global coffee prices and regulate the trade through national marketing boards who controlled the amounts of coffee supplied to the global market. The ICA, in an attempt both to secure minimum prices for producing farmers and to curb the frequent boom and bust cycle of world coffee supplies that followed sudden changes in weather patterns in producing countries (Ponte 2002). Under the ICA, state-sponsored marketing boards in exporting nations were able to withhold purchased coffee stock in times of surplus, participate in minimum price-setting agreements with outside actors, and provide quality control and processing support to domestic farmers (Kaplinsky 2004). Before its demise, the ICA and coffee boards were the principal sources of "aggregated producer power" (Kaplinsky 2004: 11) in the coffee value chain (Fridell 2007, Jaffee 2007).

When the United States withdrew from the ICA in 1989, several processes were set in motion that shaped the development of the coffee market into its current form. Coffee supplies were deregulated, marketing boards were eliminated, and coffee production was decentralized: producers who formerly aggregated their harvests through the boards now sold directly to global purchasers. The elimination of the ICA paved the way for the rise of large coffee roasting firms as the principal overseers of the "buyer-driven" value chain for coffee. Even during the ICA, the top roasters in the global coffee market had already begun consolidating control over this lucrative market through mergers and buyouts of smaller firms. For example, as early as 1960, the top four coffee roasters controlled 40 percent of all coffee sales (Pendergrast 1999: 261). The 1970s and 1980s saw similar trends; for example, the purchasing giant General Foods, owner of the Maxwell House brand, accounted for over a third of all U.S. coffee sales throughout the early part of the 1970s (Pendergrast 1999: 314).

The fall of the ICA allowed this consolidation to accelerate. By 1991, Kraft General Foods held 33 percent of the ground roasted coffee market in the United States; Procter & Gamble was close behind at 32.7 percent (Pendergrast 1999: 364). Despite the rise of gourmet coffee roasters such as Starbucks beginning in the 1990s, the vast majority of the coffee market continues to be controlled by these major roasters (Taylor 2005). By 1998, the top two international roasters controlled 49 percent of the world market share for roasted and instant coffee and the top five controlled 69 percent (Van Dijk et al. 1998 cited in Ponte 2002). By the end of the 1990s, the behemoth Nestlé controlled half of the world market for instant coffees. Once Philip Morris acquired the Maxwell House brand, it became the world's leader in roasted and ground coffees, controlling 14 percent of the entire world coffee market and 20 percent of the soluble coffee market (Pendergrast 1999: 422).

As a result of this consolidation, the contemporary international coffee trade, like that of fresh vegetables, is dominated by a few large buyers who compete with one another for small percentages of market share through careful governance of all steps in their production and supply chains. These major roasting firms in non-specialty, conventional coffee markets face a set of challenges to profit generation that are somewhat different from those in the fresh vegetable value chain. For this reason they take a different approach to supply chain governance and enforce distinct standards for coffee purchased from farmers or exporters.

Coffee is characterized by inelastic demand (Topik 2003). This means that coffee drinkers typically have a habit of daily consumption, so it is difficult for consumers to alter their purchasing pattern in reaction to price hikes or discounts. As as long ago as the postwar 1940s, spikes in coffee prices have been met with public outcry and often catch the attention of policymakers. At the same time, in the absence of ICA regulations it is increasingly difficult for roasters to maintain consistently low domestic prices for conventional coffee. Price fluctuations are much greater, subject not only to short-run changes in supplies but also to investor speculation on coffee futures (Jaffee 2007, Bacon 2005, Topik 2003). Roasters' desire to ensure cheap, ready supplies for their consumers in the face of unpredictable world pricing has led to their strategy of amassing large volumes of undifferentiated coffee beans that are regular enough to be easily substituted in and out of coffee blends without significant changes in flavor (Pendergrast 1999). For this reason, despite growing pressures from gourmet roasters offering specialty and region-specific coffees, the vast majority of the conventional coffee market remains focused on capitalizing on large supplies of lower- to medium-grade coffee varieties in an attempt to squeeze out more profits and a greater market share (Ponte and Gibbon 2005).

In sum, global production of coffee has risen with the principal aim of meeting the needs of roasters for greater volumes of uniform, lower-quality coffees. Despite continued price uncertainty, potential for oversupply of the coffee market is increasing. The 2000–2001 coffee season saw the third consecutive year in which coffee production exceeded 100 million bags (Ponte 2002). Contributing to this burgeoning supply is the entry of new coffee-producing powerhouses such as Vietnam (Ponte 2002) and farming innovations, for example the spread of higher-yielding but lower-quality African *robusta* beans, which made coffee supplies slightly more resistant to weather conditions, or sun-resistant coffee plants such as the *caturra* variety, that allows farmers to do away with shade trees that occupy valuable acreage (Pendergrast 1999: 295–296). By ensuring an environment of oversupply to the world market, roasters insulate themselves from price spikes due to weather-related shortages and offer a cheap and regular product to their consumer base.

Just as powerful supermarket chains and suppliers transferred burdens and risks to produce farmers, a small group of large, powerful roasters has ensured that coffee farmers and exporters now shoulder the burden of falling prices during periods of global oversupply and continue to face the risks of yearly price fluctuations (Ponte 2002). For farmers in non-specialty coffee markets, the options for increasing profits and insuring product quality are limited and largely out of their control. In the face of sinking conventional market prices, their only option for protecting their

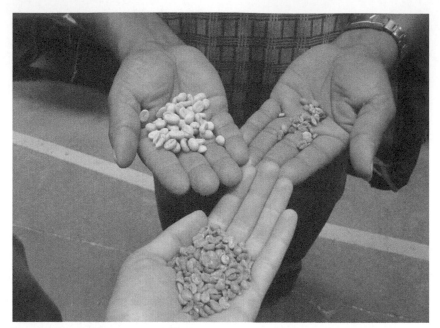

Figure 1.1.   Coffee inspection. Clockwise from upper left: *en pergamino*, as it arrives to the warehouse; defective beans selected mechanically; *oro*, high quality beans.

viability and profits is to ratchet up production and squeeze more coffee out of their landholdings. For many coffee farmers, this means embracing a new kind of agriculture that incorporates industrialized production and modern agricultural technologies.

Modern agriculture through technological innovation

The preceding sections have shown the diversity of forces impacting vegetable and coffee production chains. Coffee-production standards are driven by large-scale roasters demanding large and consistent supplies of undifferentiated coffees in a market of highly volatile prices. Vegetable standards, by contrast, are organized along a chain of "preferred suppliers" eager to consolidate large, steady volumes of produce that meet the cosmetic, safety, and quality standards of big supermarket chains. Despite these differences, both chains are characterized by power asymmetries favoring a few large-scale buyers that generate product specifications, thereby pressuring exporters who now bear a high level of risk. In response to this pressure, exporters act to condition the production processes of farmers.

Efforts to meet the demands of buyers, their standards for quality, and global circulation have centered on the application of science and technology to transcend existing environmental barriers and limitations (Murdoch and Miele 1999). In the early postwar years, the introduction of agricultural chemicals into farming systems around the world was seen as the key to securing global food supplies and agricultural commodity production (see Chapter 2). Beginning in the late 1930s and early 1940s with the discovery of the insecticidal properties of organophosphorous (OP) chemicals, soil-acting herbicides such as carbamate, and chemical-based fertilizers, a global industry emerged to solve the problem of agriculture's vulnerability to natural processes (Scott 1998, Dich et al. 1997).

As observers such as James Scott (1998) have pointed out, this process of agricultural modernization has resulted in a radical simplification of farming systems, making them more predictable and productive, as human designed technologies replace natural processes. Genetically engineered plant varieties have been substituted for naturally occurring agricultural crops, making yields more uniform and voluminous. The preferential use of chemical fertilizers over animal waste or natural soil nutrients has also made crop yields more predictable, as they are less reactive to naturally occurring variations in soil fertilities. Finally, the use of herbicides, fungicides, and insecticides has helped to secure optimal conditions for crops to produce yields that are uniform in shape, size, and maturity.

Epidemiology of pesticide exposure

The apparent advances brought by modern agricultural technologies were soon met with growing concerns about the negative effects of the global agrochemical trade on public health. Scientific advances in the 1940s and 1950s made it possible to track the health effects of exposure to smaller quantities of chemicals, fueling national and international attempts to regulate the chemical trade. Specifically, the development of research techniques and technologies for detecting smaller quantities of chemicals in organisms and the environment allowed researchers to identify the impacts of exposure using microbiological endpoints. In this new era of "minipollutant" research (Buccini 2004), studies increasingly questioned the safety of established and widely used pesticide ingredients such as arsenic and mercury compounds, organochlorine and OP compounds, atrazine, and other chemicals (see Sanborn et al. 2004 for a review of case studies from the past three decades).

Many agrochemical pesticides gradually have been phased out of circulation because of the established risks that they present to human health and the environment. However, a lack of consensus persists within the scientific community regarding the actual effects of many agrochemical ingredients that are still widely used. This then slows any attempt at enacting policy in the interests of protecting those exposed to such ingredients. It is clear that pesticides work by intentionally attacking one or more physical aspects of unwanted pests, such as insects or fungi. However, establishing a correlation between suspected adverse health effects and exposure to these agrochemicals, particularly among human populations, is difficult. Still being debated are many of the potential health effects of agricultural pesticides and other crop treatments on farmers, applicators, greenhouse workers, chemical factory employees, or any other individuals coming into contact with such substances. Although numerous epidemiological studies have established statistically significant correlations between exposure to a given chemical and adverse health effects, a direct causal relationship and causal mechanisms are much harder to establish. Pesticide exposure has been statistically and circumstantially linked to a range of short-term acute health effects such as nausea, dizziness, and nervous system damage, as well as numerous effects of long-term exposure such as certain forms of cancer, tumor development, neurodegenerative disease, and reproductive or hormonal disorders. At the same time, a many studies investigating the link between pesticide exposure and adverse health conditions have been unable to isolate a precise cause-and-effect relationship. Despite the fact that the existence of contradictory evidence in no way invalidates the assertion that there is a correlation between exposure to certain agrochemicals and the appearance of adverse health outcomes, it is this direct causal link between one particular chemical and a precise physiological outcome that is most often required as a basis for implementing protective policy.

This body of research often fails to produce unequivocal results for a number of reasons. First, researchers face unavoidable challenges in framing the subjects in question—defining pesticide exposure and isolating populations exposed to a given chemical. In the realm of occupational exposure, a broad spectrum of populations with highly varied levels of exposure have been considered, including farmers (Smit et al. 2003, Rohlman et al. 2001, Cole et al. 1997, London et al. 1997), pesticide applicators (Farahat et al. 2003, Daniell et al. 1992), farmworkers (Kamel et al. 2003, Recio et al. 2001, Engel et al. 1998), greenhouse workers (Roldán-Tapia et al. 2005, Bazylewicz-Walczak et al. 1999, Nehez et al. 1988), and pesticide chemical factory workers (Padungtod et al. 1999, Jabloniká et al. 1989). Adding to this diversity of occupational class, an array of agrochemical mixes to which each class may be exposed gives rise to highly varied and contradictory results within even this small group of studies.

Outside the occupational realm, studies concerning the health risks of pesticide exposure among specific population segments also render often-contradictory results. Studies have focused on the specific health effects of exposure among women (Fieten et al. 2009), children (Daniels et al. 1997), single ethnic groups (Dosemeci et al. 1994), and populations from a broad range of geographies (Miranda et al. 2002, Wesseling et al. 2002, Cole et al. 1997). The varied findings associated with each different population segment add yet another layer of complexity to efforts at establishing a causal connection between chemical exposure and a given health outcome.

A second factor that contributes to diverging results across epidemiological studies is the sheer number of chemicals to which an individual may be exposed. It is rare that an individual, farmer or otherwise, is regularly exposed to a single, isolated chemical. Commonly applied pesticides are mixtures of numerous potentially hazardous chemical compounds. The challenge of identifying the effects of a single chemical is heightened by the fact that farmers tend to vary the chemicals they apply either annually or by season. As one review points out, "There are over 400 different pesticide chemicals approved for use in agriculture, which might be formulated into thousands of different products available for users. Farmers may use dozens of different chemicals over a season and they may vary from season to season" (Hanke and Jurewicz 2004: 239). This situation obfuscates attempts to establish a causal link between a health outcome and one among potentially hundreds of chemicals to which an individual may be exposed. Further, it introduces a series of underlying variables and potential interaction effects between chemicals that give rise to seemingly contradictory results across epidemiological studies.

A third factor contributing to the lack of consensus surrounding the human health effects of pesticide exposure is the diversity of methodologies and metrics employed by existing epidemiological studies, preventing researchers from accurately comparing their findings. Definitions of exposure vary widely across studies. Researchers investigating the effects of even a single chemical have gauged exposure to pesticides by focusing on farmer application technique and knowledge of safety practices (Gomes et al. 1999), site of exposure (Fenske 1997), type of protective equipment used when spraying (Hines et al. 2001), or type of crop sprayed (London and Myers 1998). In other cases, researchers have employed proxy measures of pesticide exposure ranging from a history of high exposure levels (Wesseling et al. 2002), holding an occupation determined to be at high risk for exposure (London et al. 1997), or even residence in a rural area where chemicals are commonly sprayed (Cole et al. 1997). High variation in the way that each study defines exposure makes comparison problematic: as one review points out, "The link between these classifications and the actual exposure is often unknown, and it is possible that the amount of exposure in any given population varies considerably" (McCauley et al. 2006: 956).

Beyond the methodological issue of defining exposure levels of experimental groups, studies considering similar classes of health effects and chemical compounds also demonstrate a wide range of approaches for detecting such effects. For example, in a review focusing on the neurobehavioral effects of populations exposed to a popular class of pesticides containing organophosphates (OP), McCauley et al. (2006) report the use of seven different test batteries among studies conducted within the span of twelve years. Tests employed included the World Health Organization Neurobehavioral Core Test Battery (NCTB), the Wechsler Adult Intelligence Scale (WAIS-R), and the Neurobehavioral Evaluation System (NES). These reviewed studies rendered highly varied results, even among those employing the same test (see Reidy et al. 1992, and Rosenstock et al. 1991). In studies of the potential cancer-causing effects of various pesticides and pesticide mixtures, even the use of biomarkers such as the presence of a chromosomal aberration or micronuclei do not ensure consensus across studies (see Bolognesi 2003 for a review). Overall, among epidemiological studies of the health effects of pesticides, the high degree of variation in methodology, in indicators of pesticide exposure and risk, and in metrics employed for gauging the outcomes of exposure make establishing a link to any health outcome extremely difficult.

Human health effects of acute and long-term agrochemical exposure: the case of organophosphate pesticides

In spite of contradictory evidence, a large body of research *has* established links between several major health risks and exposure to ingredients in commonly circulated pesticides. Epidemiological research typically has focused on two principal types of chemical exposure that have the potential to affect human health in different ways: acute pesticide poisoning and longer-term exposure to low or medium levels of pesticides.

Acute pesticide poisoning occurs when a person is exposed in a single instance to high levels of toxic chemicals, causing immediate health consequences for the individual. Documented effects of acute pesticide poisoning include minor symptoms such as dizziness, headache, and fatigue as well as more serious impacts such as blurred vision, neurological impairment, respiratory depression, seizures, paralysis, and death (PAN

2010). A widely cited report by the WHO (2004) estimates that three million acute pesticide poisonings occur annually around the globe, resulting in 250,000 deaths. The majority of these deaths are due to *intentional* exposure and suicide, but the data are widely criticized for being too conservative and failing to account for the magnitude of unreported cases of *unintentional* exposure (Murray et al. 2002, Jeyaratnam 1990).

While the range of studies concerning the effects of acute exposure to different pesticide ingredients is extremely broad in scope, the case of OP pesticides (used in the highly popular but recently restricted product Tamaron), one of the most commonly used pesticide classes in Guatemala (Hurst 1999), is illustrative. The toxicity of OP pesticides is derived from the fact that they inhibit the body's production of the chemical erythrocyte acetylcholinesterase, which regulates brain and nervous system functioning. Less severe symptoms of acute OP poisoning in humans include headaches, nausea, and vomiting; more severe poisoning induces muscle weakness, heart rate changes, coma, and death (Kamel and Hoppin 2004, Ecobichon 2001). Several studies (Miranda et al. 2002, Wesseling et al. 2002, London et al. 1998) have confirmed the connection between acute OP pesticide poisoning and these symptoms and have shown that symptoms persist in humans long after the instance of initial exposure (see Kamel and Hoppin 2004 for a review).

There is a high level of consensus surrounding the data linking these symptoms to acute OP pesticide exposure (McCauley et al. 2006, Keifer and Mahurin 1997). Less consensus exists concerning the data on health effects of exposure to medium and lower amounts of OP chemical mixtures over time. One reason is the increasing difficulty of isolating the effects of a single chemical over time, as individuals are exposed a greater number of chemical mixtures with each passing season. Research is also complicated by underreporting of chemical poisoning when individuals do not seek medical attention for exposure-related symptoms (Calvert et al. 2003). Even when an individual does seek medical attention, symptoms are frequently misdiagnosed by medical personnel, who often have no specialized training in the diagnosis of pesticide poisoning (National Environmental Education and Training Foundation 2002). Many studies attempt to overcome reporting problems by using biomarkers to determine levels of exposure for studied populations. However, unlike organochloride chemicals, OP pesticides have a relatively short half-life, leaving only a limited amount of time between actual exposure to the chemical and the disappearance of appropriate indicators in an individual's body (McCauley et al. 2006: 956). Finally, estimating the level of exposure of a given individual is complicated by the variation in experiences with agrochemicals a person may have had over time. For example, many people have diverse work histories, so the current use of safety equipment does not necessarily reflect access to such protections across employment scenarios over time. Farm workers in particular tend to have a wide range of experiences farming many types of crops, some requiring more chemical applications, others requiring fewer. While recording occupational histories for study participants can offer clues to researchers concerning the relative level of agrochemical exposure, designing experimental groups based on participants' ability to recall the exact circumstances of their contact with different chemicals is often problematic.

This complexity of practices makes producing conclusive evidence of the effects of specific chemicals on quantifiable health indicators a difficult task. In the case of OP pesticides, despite a substantial amount of contradictory evidence, long-term exposure to this class of chemical has been tied by numerous studies to low performance on neurobehavioral test batteries (Kamel and Hoppin 2004, Farahat et al. 2003); decreased scores on measures of cognitive performance (Korsak and Sato 1977); certain types of neurodegenerative disease (Bhatt et al. 1999, Seidler et al. 1996); specific reproductive disorders (Hanke and Jurewicz 2004, Recio et al. 2001, Curtis et al. 1999, Savitz et al. 1997); and some forms of cancer (Bolognesi 2003, Padmavathi et al. 2000, Kourakis et al. 1992). Further, according to a review by Kamel and Hoppin (2004: 952) concerning pesticide exposure and prevalence of a host of symptoms, "Most studies have focused on OPs; most of these found an association of exposure with increased symptom prevalence."

Again, it is true that several studies have produced evidence to the contrary. Concerning the connection between pesticide exposure and neurobehavioral performance, one review points out, "fourteen studies examining pesticide exposure included a variant of the digit span test [a test of memory most popularly used as a part of the Wechsler Adult Intelligence Scale (WAIS)]. Of these studies comparing exposed populations (defined by exposure or by occupational group), four showed significant deficits between exposed and control populations, four showed decrements in performance related to exposure, and six showed no decrements in performance" (McCauley et al. 2006: 956). Several studies (e.g., Chancellor et al. 1993, Granieri et al. 1988) failed to find any evidence to support the connection between OP exposure and neurodegenerative disease. Reporting on potential reproductive effects of OP exposure, reviewers Hanke and Jurewicz (2004: 225) indicate that the case for a direct connection between exposure to pesticides and difficulty conceiving children was supported by only three out of seven studies conducted in European

countries. Finally, in a 2003 review of the genotoxicity of pesticide exposure, Bolognesi (2003) echoes the conclusion of many studies by arguing
that the link between pesticide exposure and cancer is highly conditioned
by the degree of exposure. She concludes, "The cytogenetic damage in-
duced by pesticides appears to depend on the degree of exposure. A dose-
response relationship can be hypothesized. Negative results have been
associated with low levels of exposure. By contrast, clearly positive results were reported in populations subject to high exposure levels, namely
people suffering from severe [acute] intoxication" (Bolognesi 2003: 267).
Overall, the evidence presented in these studies seems to directly contra-
dict or, at least, complicate the findings of those establishing a correlation
between human exposure to OP pesticides and detrimental health effects,
making it difficult to establish or implement protective regulation.

The heightened risk of pesticide exposure in Central America

Because the level of chemical exposure affects the severity of health outcomes, many studies highlight the importance of farmer education about
the toxicity of various agrochemicals, the use of safety equipment, and
proper handling procedures. However, access to information and protective equipment is often limited, particularly in the developing world,
where pesticide monitoring institutions and organizations can be weak or
nonexistent.

In the case of OP pesticides, while studies (Maizlish et al. 1987,
Dick et al. 2001) found no significant connections between exposure to
OP pesticides among "well-trained and -equipped pesticide applicators
in the United States" (Kamel and Hoppin 2004: 952), several studies conducted in the developing world found increased prevalence of symptoms
for neurotoxicity among several groups exposed to OPs (Ohayo-Mitoko
et al. 2000, London et al. 1998). In this case, diverging results may be related to higher degrees of pesticide exposure of workers in the developing
world due to lack of proper training or access to safety equipment. For
example, in the case of Guatemalan coffee workers, recent survey results
indicate that, among commercial coffee farms using agrochemicals, only
9 percent provide protective equipment for workers in the coffee-growing
Department of Huehuetenango and only 35 percent do so in the Department of Jalapa (Castillejos et al. 2010). Nationwide, where approximately
7 percent of the country's population (Gresser and Tickell 2002: 8) of
13 million (Bowser and Mahal 2010) work in coffee, the number of coffee workers performing their job without adequate equipment may range
from approximately 82,000 to 318,500.

However, lack of safety equipment or education in the use of potentially toxic agrochemicals is only one of many factors contributing to increased risk of adverse health effects related to agrochemical exposure for farmers in the developing world. As Smith et al. (2008) point out, many classes of chemicals that are either unregistered or severely restricted in their countries of origin are exported to developing nations that have weaker restrictions or less ability to enforce existing agrochemical regulations. According to a study conducted between 2001 and 2003, Guatemala was the fifth largest importer of pesticides designated by the U.S. Code of Federal Regulations as Class I, the most highly toxic pesticides (Smith et al. 2008: 171). Weak regulatory mechanisms and lax monitoring of agrochemical circulation at the national level prevent governments in recipient countries such as Guatemala from being able to adequately assess or respond to health problems experienced by populations exposed to toxic pesticides within their borders.

This issue is exacerbated by the fact that, in most cases, exposed individuals in the developing world do not seek medical attention for symptoms related to pesticide exposure. Unlike farmers in developed nations, farmers in agricultural export regions such as Central America are often exposed to pesticides in rural areas that can be long distances from the nearest medical facility. Even when care is accessible, most small farmers or agricultural workers in Central America lack the basic economic resources to afford adequate medical attention. For these and other reasons, it is likely that opting not to seek medical attention for exposure-related illness is the rule rather than the exception. According to survey data from the early 2000s, Murray et al. (2002: 243) estimate that rates of underreporting of pesticide-related illness among Central American farmers is as high as 98%.

In Guatemala specifically, researchers have argued that there are between four and six unreported cases of pesticide exposure for every one in which an individual seeks medical attention (Hurst 1999). Even when farmers seek medical attention for symptoms related to pesticide exposure in the developing world, their conditions are frequently misdiagnosed by clinic staff, who often lack sufficient training for identifying exposure-related symptoms (Connan 1996). This problem is particularly severe for women, who are less likely to be accurately diagnosed with pesticide poisoning (London et al. 2002). Observing this specific combination of weak regulatory and surveillance mechanisms at the national level, lack of farmer education and access to safety equipment, rising levels of national consumption of restricted agrochemical classes, and inadequate medical treatment infrastructures, Murray et al. (2002: 243) refer to

Central America as a "world leader in pesticide use and pesticide-related problems."

Efforts to regulate agrochemical circulation

While many regulatory bodies and industry leaders continue to wait for uncontested epidemiological evidence linking specific agrochemicals to a set of outcomes in human health, other international bodies have already taken measures to protect at-risk farming populations, particularly in the developing world. In the absence of unanimous and converging data concerning the effects of agrochemicals on the health of human populations, many national and international regulators turn to the results of studies of chemical exposure in lab animals. The major organizations that classify chemicals according to the risks they present to humans—the United States Environmental Protection Agency (EPA)'s Office of Pesticide Programs, the United States National Institutes of Health (NIH), the UN's FAO and WHO, and the International Agency for Research on Cancer (IARC)—therefore rank individual chemicals on spectrums based on the possible and probable risks they pose to human populations using a combination of evidence from lab animals and epidemiological research (PAN 2003). These rankings form the base upon which national and international regulatory frameworks for agrochemicals historically have been built.

Though many countries, particularly those in the global north, had already enacted some form of agrochemical regulation by the 1950s (Buccini 2004), the 1970s and the decades to follow saw a surge of international agreements formed to curb the circulation of chemicals known or suspected to threaten public health. One of the earliest efforts to enlist the cooperation of national governments occurred in 1985 with the drafting of the International Code of Conduct on the Distribution and Use of Pesticides by the WHO and FAO. This voluntary code targeted developing countries by outlining a regulatory framework and procedures for disseminating information concerning safe handling of chemicals suspected to be toxic (FAO 2002).

Several major milestones for global pesticide regulation came later in the 1990s in the wake of the 1992 UN Conference on Environment and Development (UNCED) in Rio de Janeiro (Buccini 2004). One significant result of the UNCED effort was a new focus on international sales of chemicals that were severely restricted or banned in their countries of origin, primarily the United States and Europe. Despite the fact that many such chemicals cannot be sold in the countries in which they were produced, restrictions rarely exist on the sales of banned chemicals to developing countries that have no restrictive regulations. This loophole allows surplus stockpiles of banned chemicals to accumulate in importing countries.

The Rotterdam Convention of the FAO and UNEP attempts to address this issue by preventing the import of hazardous chemicals into developing nations. The convention went into effect in 1998 and has since been signed by over 150 nations. Among the treaty's contents is a ban of twenty-two specific pesticides through a system of Prior Informed Consent (PIC). The PIC system aims to provide information and a process for making decisions to importing nations concerning the effective regulation or restriction of pesticides known to pose threats to public health. The convention also contains provisions for enlisting the efforts of exporting countries to prevent shipments of banned chemicals to participating nations in the developing world (UNEP 2012).

Similar to Rotterdam's PIC system, the Stockholm Convention of the UNEP and FAO attempts to limit the spread of specific agricultural chemicals, labeled Persisting Organic Pollutants (POPs). This 2001 agreement started with the "Dirty Dozen," a priority list of twelve chemicals, and has since been expanded to eliminate the circulation of additional chemicals found to present serious risks to human health. Through its Intergovernmental Negotiating Committee, the Stockholm agreement attempts to enact a full ban on POPs by requiring member nations to enact regulatory measures that prevent their production and spread, promote public awareness of the threats of POPs through educational programs, and monitor their use within their borders (Buccini 2004).

The efforts of the Stockholm and Rotterdam conventions have met with major successes across the globe. Apart from securing written compliance and national pesticide regulation plans from over 130 national governments, their strategy of targeting specific chemicals won widespread bans on many of the worst toxic pesticides, such as chlordane, dieldrin, heptachlor, and mirex. As a result of the Stockholm Convention, the Global Alliance for Alternatives to DDT was formed and held its first conference on April 26, 2011 (UNEP n.d.).

Loopholes in agrochemical regulation

Despite these major successes in global regulation, pesticides remain a problem throughout much of the developing world. The majority of pesticide poisonings occur in the developing world and a large percentage is comprised of unintentional, occupational exposure in agriculture. To understand why pesticides continue to pose significant health threats to farming populations in spite of international efforts, we must look more closely at how international agreements such as the Rotterdam Convention are designed and enforced.

First, many international conventions are completely voluntary and therefore subject to the political will of national governments. For example, the UNEP Stockholm Convention concerning POPs has not been ratified by the United States, the largest exporter of agrochemicals in the Western Hemisphere (UNEP 2004). Many pesticides banned for use in countries such as the United States can still be exported to developing nations, regardless of international restriction. According to Smith et al. (2008), between 2001 and 2003 alone, over 28 million pounds of pesticides banned in the United States left the country's ports. Pesticides classified by WHO as "extremely hazardous," Class Ia chemicals, left U.S. ports at an average of 16 tons per day. During this period, an estimated half billion pounds of pesticides known to cause cancer were exported.

Second, even when national governments opt to participate in international regulatory agreements, the degree to which they enforce treaty provisions is often influenced by external interests. For example, consultation with chemical industry stakeholders has been a growing trend in international chemical agreements under the UN. The recognition that the problem of harmful chemical circulation requires partnerships not only between regulators and nations but also agrochemical industry leaders has prompted the formation of many initiatives that seek greater involvement of key industry stakeholders. Of course, industry partners tend to have an economic interest in minimizing restriction of their own products, and their participation may lead to weaker agreements. For example, the FAO's International Code of Conduct, largely drafted in conjunction with the global pesticide industry organization, Global Crop Protection Federation, has been criticized for failing to include "mandatory or enforceable reductions in the use of the most hazardous pesticides" as a result of the federation's influence (Murray and Taylor 2000: 1737).

Particular regions and areas of the globe are more affected by toxic chemicals than others. Within the developing world, Latin American nations stand apart for elevated risk to public health from toxic agrochemicals. Over the past several decades, the total share of pesticides consumed by Latin America has spiked from 9 percent of world pesticide consumption in 1985 to 21 percent in 2008 (PAN 2010: 4). Throughout the region, increasing rates of pesticide consumption and domestic production combine with a lack of national resources and human capital to enforce regulations. The result is a situation in which the public health of millions of people is endangered in spite of attempts by their governing institutions to participate in international regulatory agreements.

Even among Latin American countries, Guatemala stands out as an area for concern. Production and export of crops such as coffee and fresh vegetables has made the agricultural sector a powerhouse of the country's economy. Among Guatemala's approximately 1.2 million farmers and agricultural workers, around 80 percent are regularly exposed to pesticides through their work (Hurst 1999: 8-9). Of these pesticides, a high proportion are either severely restricted or known to be toxic. Between 2001 and 2003, Guatemala was the fifth largest recipient of WHO Class I toxins leaving U.S. ports (Smith et al. 2008: 171). Approximately 80 percent of insecticides entering the country contain carbamate and OP compounds, two highly toxic classes of chemical that are suspected to present hazards to the human nervous system (Hurst 1999). A large number of these pesticides are destined for use by farmers of fresh vegetables (Thrupp et al. 1995) and coffee, the world's third-most sprayed crop following cotton and tobacco (Pendergrast 1999: 398).

High volumes of pesticide coming into the nation meet with an extremely weak regulatory regime and low levels of government involvement in worker protection. In Guatemala, three major governmental ministries are involved in one or more aspects of chemical pesticide regulation: the Ministries of Health, of Agriculture and Livestock, and of Economy. While there exist numerous national decrees regarding the registration, use, and circulation of chemicals within the country, efforts at coordinating at the national and local levels are often thwarted by lack of resources and capabilities within the involved ministries. National efforts to control pesticides are weakened by lack of political will or competing interests. The push to liberalize trade in agrochemicals is in constant tension with efforts to regulate. Further, global pesticide industry groups such as CropLife International (formerly GIFAP, GCPF) are frequently involved in the country's national efforts to control pesticides, raising concerns about the effectiveness of resulting policies (Murray and Taylor 2000).

Here, the case of one of the country's largest efforts to promote farmer safety, the Global Safe Use Campaign, is illustrative (Murray and Taylor 2000). With the influence of industry organizations such as CropLife International, the program emphasized farmer education rather than direct control or regulation of agrochemicals. Training several hundreds of thousands of farmers in safe use of pesticides and protective equipment in the first years following the program's start in 1991, pesticide industry sponsors touted the success of the initiative (Murray and Taylor 2000). However, the data presented by organizers as evidence of increased safety of Guatemalan farmers were subsequently criticized (see Murray and Taylor 2000, Hurst 1999) for proclaiming a decrease in reports of pesticide poisonings in areas where the entire health care system had coincidentally been brought to a halt due to a bloody civil war (see Murray and Taylor 2000, Hurst 1999). These critics argue that drops in pesticide use among Guatemalan farmers reported by leaders of the program's campaign largely can be attributed to the collapse of the country's cotton industry, a notoriously chemical-intense form of agriculture (Murray and Taylor 2000). Such critics counter that estimates of pesticide poisonings in Guatemala are systematically low, due to underreporting and failure of many poisoned individuals to seek medical attentions. Research among Guatemalan vegetable growers has in fact revealed high instances of reported overuse of chemical pesticides, applications of pesticides without proper safety equipment, and misunderstandings concerning the effects of many pesticides on human health (Hamilton and Fischer 2003, Arbona 1998). More recent estimates of pesticide poisonings claim rates as high as ten thousand annually in some of Guatemala's agricultural regions (Murray and Taylor 2000: 1793).

Beyond regulation: agrochemical misuse and abuse

Beyond the lapses in effectiveness of public and private efforts to regulate pesticides in Guatemala and the pressures on farmers to produce large amounts of export crops according to purchaser specifications, there remain several fundamental barriers to reducing the risk of pesticide exposure at the farm level. Major issues identified by researchers include lack of access to or failure to use proper safety equipment (Matthew 2008), farmer credit systems that make agrochemical purchases a prerequisite for loans (Murray and Taylor 2000), and lack of sufficient knowledge among farmers of safe handling procedures for toxic chemicals (Arbona 1998).

However, as we will show in this book, the problem of toxic pesticide use and exposure is often rooted in something more profound than simple misunderstanding. We found that many farmers in Guatemala knew very well the risks posed by their use of chemical pesticides. Their view of the inevitability of chemical use frequently paralleled a well-established concept called the "agricultural treadmill." First detailed in 1958 by agricultural economist Willard Cochrane, the treadmill of agricultural production affects farmers as they adopt new technologies such as agrochemicals to increase the outputs of the crops they grow. The technologies that farmers purchase have the short-term effect of allowing early adopters to produce a crop such as coffee or vegetables more intensively per season, making it possible for them to sell more, creating the illusion of a greater sustained profit. However, as more farmers begin to adopt new technologies over time, markets suffer from surpluses of products that outstrip existing demand. This forces prices down. Farmers are then faced with lower selling prices for their crops and higher investments in new, state of the art technologies. As incomes fall, farmers have little choice but to buy the newest farm inputs in order to stay ahead of declining market prices. Greater production then leads to significant drops in prices, setting in motion a treadmill effect that keeps farmers dependent upon the new, potentially dangerous agricultural products in order to keep farming profitable.

This combination of export market structures, purchaser quality standards, porous regulatory frameworks, and Cochrane's agricultural treadmill keeps farmers using many chemicals that they know pose significant threats to their health. Though in our research many farmers made reference to the bind of falling market prices for their goods and increased costs of new technologies, they also described several other ways in which the inertia of toxic chemical use is perpetuated. In Chapters Four and Five, we explore these socioeconomic influences in greater detail through the eyes of small coffee and vegetable producing farmers in the Guatemalan countryside. But first, the next chapter details the ways in which agrochemical use differentially affects specific groups. Highlighting key structural, economic, and cultural patterns, it will demonstrate how some people are more vulnerable than others to the health threats of persistent agrochemical use.

Chapter 2

Public Health and
Vulnerable Populations

Agriculture is a source of livelihood for billions of people around the world and is of particular economic importance in the developing world. We have shown that the global economy has had a tremendous impact on the experience of agricultural workers the world over, and producers around the globe find themselves racing one another to earn a profit, competing in the only means available to them: producing more and selling faster. In the 1960s, the Green Revolution promised to alleviate poverty for farmers in the form of advanced agricultural chemicals and diffusion of technological innovation (Grübler 2003). From the 1970s to the 1990s, the promise of integration into the global economy encouraged national governments of developing countries to pursue agricultural expansion into previously uncultivated land (Berger 1992). Finally, the global market that grew out of trade liberalization of the 1990s allowed freer international circulation of goods, so farmers were able to intensify their production by planting high-yield seed varieties, applying fertilizers that allowed plants to grow larger and faster, and spraying plants with pesticides to minimize crop losses (Hogstedt et al. 2007, Matson et al. 1997).

A global economy means that corporations can source labor in any country, city, or village willing to accept their business. This is advantageous to multinational corporations who seek to minimize costs of production by relocating in constant pursuit of ever-lower labor costs. But as national governments continue to lower safety and environmental restrictions in an effort to attract corporate investments, these changes have taken a toll on the public health of workers in developing countries, who are less likely to have formal training in safe work practices and less apt to register complaints regarding unsafe working conditions. The flexible labor pool that fills these temporary and seasonal employment opportunities is often comprised of women and children, who are particularly vulnerable to the dangers of agrochemical exposure.

The rapid expansion of opportunities to produce and sell goods globally has led farmers to take increasing risks to personal, family, community, and international safety in order to remain competitive. For example, while technological advances such as industrialized agriculture boost production, social theorists such as Ulrich Beck (1992) and Anthony Giddens (1990) have argued that they also carry exponentially heightened risks and safety concerns for producers and consumers alike. For example, we know that where farmers have greater access to chemical products but insufficient information about product safety, vendors tend to promote—and uninformed farmers tend to follow—a "more is better" application philosophy, resulting in ever-higher costs of production, greater dependence on chemical inputs, and graver threats to global public health (Corriols Molina 2009, Guidotti and Gitterman 2007, Hogstedt et al. 2007, Mull and Kirkhorn 2005, Mathews et al. 2003, Popper et al. 1996). And when farmers allocate a greater amount of crops to export sales than family consumption, dietary diversity in rural households is diminished, exacerbating already high malnutrition rates in the developing world (Hogstedt et al. 2007).

In Guatemala in particular, a perfect storm of global, national, and local conditions has rendered agricultural commodity producers both cripplingly dependent on the use of pesticides and exceptionally vulnerable to the ill effects of pesticide exposure. This chapter reviews the literature on global public health to demonstrate how a complex mélange of inadequate public services, low levels of education, high rates of malnutrition, and extreme poverty places all classes of agricultural workers in developing countries—and in Guatemala, particularly rural, indigenous, and clandestine working populations—at heightened risk of pesticide poisoning.

International development and the "immiseration" of public health services

Farmers frequently intensify agricultural production with the assistance of state leaders. When the Washington Consensus was established in 1989, global economic leadership encouraged developing nations to become better competitors in the international economy through greater investment in the activities in which they hold a comparative advantage. These advantages generally take the form of abundant arable land and a mobile labor pool of workers who can enter the workforce when needed for economic growth and leave the workforce when jobs become scarce (Chenery 1961). As a result, the late 1970s and early 1980s saw countries of the developing world borrowing hundreds of millions of dollars from international lending institutions such as International Monetary Fund (IMF) and World Bank in order to invest in the development of their specialized national economies.

The economic policies that guide the lending practices of the IMF and World Bank view greater market integration as a primary goal of developing countries (Stiglitz 2004). As a condition of their loans, then, borrowing countries have to demonstrate a plan for repayment, usually including provisions to generate more revenue by attracting the business of foreign companies. Lending institutions assist in the design of repayment plans, called Structural Adjustment Policies, which commonly feature capital market liberalization policies to create a more attractive environment for investors (Stiglitz 2004). In effect, "capital market liberalization" means national governments are asked to loosen regulations on corporations and business practices, including restrictions on environmental responsibility and worker safety and weaken the power of trade unions. Protections for workers and the environment are important for human and environmental health, but are opposed by the transnational corporations that development nations want to attract because these regulations often translate into additional production costs—such as water treatment, hazardous material equipment, and safety training.

It is because of these loosened restrictions on the flow of goods as well as relaxed environmental protections that agrochemicals that have been banned or severely restricted in high-income countries continue to circulate freely in the developing world (Hogstedt et al. 2007). In 1995, the WHO estimated that 50–100 percent of workers in developing countries who are employed in industries such as agriculture and manufacturing were exposed to hazardous materials beyond the exposure limits permitted in industrialized countries (cited in Hogstedt et al. 2007). Moreover, another hallmark of structural adjustment is the tendency to siphon money from social program budgets and redirect these funds toward loan repayment (Rudel 2007, Collier and Gunning 1999). In sum, the terms of international borrowing agreements have pressured governments in the developing world to spend less in the areas of health care and education, while removing environmental and safety regulations at the same time that families are working harder and intensifying agricultural production.

While vigorous debate has weighed the positive and negative short-run effects of structural adjustment on economic growth and development (see OECD 2011, Pfeiffer and Chapman 2010, Stiglitz 2002, Dollar and Svensson 2000, Sparr 1994, Summers and Pritchett 1993), anthropologists on the ground have witnessed what Pfeiffer and Chapman (2010) call the "immiseration" of individuals and households resulting from market liberalization and cuts to public health spending. Structural adjustment policies are likely to escalate existing public health concerns in developing countries in many ways, for example by:

- Cutting budgets for public sector health care
- Imposing fees and removing subsidies for public services such as clinics and transportation
- Cutting budgets to infrastructural support such as education, sanitation, water treatment, and agricultural subsidies
- Reducing access to health care by cutting public sector employment, resulting in massive layoffs and financial hardship
- Devaluing national currency which results in price increases for basic needs (Breman and Shelton 2007)

Consequently, producers in heavily indebted countries are particularly vulnerable to the ill effects of agrochemical exposure, as they are poorly prepared to identify and treat symptoms and unequipped to cease chemical application.

In defense of public sector reductions under structural adjustment policies, researchers working for the IMF have argued that increases in public spending will not be sufficient to improve health outcomes in recipient countries where the government is generally ineffective (Gupta et al. 2002). They also highlight the role of governmental corruption in producing negative public health outcomes from a number of angles. Because corruption is frequently associated with higher military spending and lower spending on health and education, it provokes higher prices for public services and lowers the quality of service available, which discourages the public from accessing the health care they need and reduces the willingness of the public to pay taxes, thereby reducing the government revenue available for investment in human capital.

Similarly, corruption, mismanagement, and absenteeism in the developing world are seen as "market failures," and as a result, when the health care system is plagued by such market failures, the neoliberal economic policies promoted by IMF and World Bank are rendered ineffective (Lewis 2006). Market strategies to promote competition and improve services in health care systems in the developing world are not been effective because, researchers argue, undereducated populations are ill prepared to evaluate their health care options. In short, primary health care programs have met with limited success because the amount of money spent in health care is immaterial when efficacy of government systems is low.

Filmer et al. emphasize, "Readers in industrial countries without personal experience may find it difficult to appreciate just how poor the quality of public sector services can be" (2000: 208). Indeed, despite well-intended efforts to provide health care access at a variety of levels and locations, in practice, the system is often a shadow of its carefully planned self.

All of these conditions describe the situation in Guatemala, a country with a total population of around 13 million, or about one third of the population of Central America (Bowser and Mahal 2010). According to the World Bank, in 2011 Guatemala's external debt (owed to IMF and other lending agencies) exceeded US$16 trillion (World Bank n.d.a). While the Guatemalan economy was described in 2003 as the largest in Central America (Gragnolati and Marini 2003), the United Nations Development Report indicates that the country's government dedicated the second smallest share of its gross domestic product (GDP) to public spending on health (1.9 percent) among Latin American countries (Bowser and Mahal 2010). Guatemala has long been plagued by an ineffective government, which hinders the allocation of public funds to vital sectors such as public health. In 2010, an investigation by the International Commission Against Impunity in Guatemala (CICIG), an international body created by the UN in 2006 to investigate clandestine security organizations committing human rights violations (CICIG n.d.), resulted in arrest warrants for nineteen officials accused of carrying out "continuous criminal activity involving killings, drug trafficking, money laundering, kidnappings, extortions and drug robberies" (Maya 2010). These officials held some of the highest offices in the country, from the Ministry of Government to the National Civil Police.

The "immiseration" of health care in Guatemala

As a result of the combination of cuts to public spending and misappropriation of government funds, Guatemala's public health care system in practice bears little resemblance to the comprehensive structure intended by the Ministry of Public Health and Social Assistance. Ideally, community health centers and health posts are accessible at the "town" level (Weller et al. 1997). Community health centers are the simplest health facilities, staffed by volunteers and visited monthly by doctors and health technicians. Health posts are government-run health facilities, staffed by an auxiliary nurse and a health technician, providing preventive and primary health care (Gragnolati and Marini 2003). Attesting to the strain on these public facilities, Ron's 1999 study of health insurance in Guatemala and the Philippines found that indigenous rural areas were typically served by one health center and one health post, staffed by one physician, three nurses, one pharmacist, ten auxiliary nurses, and twenty health promoters, all serving a population of more than sixty-five thousand people. In Guatemala City, by contrast, one doctor serves around six hundred residents. Beyond the town level, private clinics and hospitals are located in cities. While some basic services were still provided free of charge in hospitals, fees had been newly introduced for routine health needs such as diagnostic procedures and lab work.

Our research found these services to be even sparer than projected in Ron's 1999 report. In one coffee growing community, a doctor came to visit the health center only once in fifteen months. He occupied the community eco-lodge to service a line of more than one hundred residents who lined up at dawn for the rare opportunity to have their blood sugar checked and inquire about various ailments—chronic headaches, hernias, Hepatitis A, a lump in the breast, and so on. Another community had a health center that opened regularly to service community residents as well as visitors from a number of neighboring villages, but the volunteer staff complained that they had not received sufficient training to treat properly the most common ailments experienced by the community. Volunteer workers also complained that their supplies were meager and useless; indeed, the shelves were stocked arbitrarily—acetaminophen, tampons, cold medicine, three one-month packs of birth control pills. Volunteers were in desperate need of the most basic supplies for cleaning and treating wounds such as cuts and burns, anti-diarrheal medications, and antibiotics. Similarly, among six vegetable-growing communities in which we have worked, only two public clinics—one equipped with a steady flow of volunteer workers and one permanently staffed with a nurse—were available to serve the entire population of 908 households with an average of 6.6 persons per family.

The poor quality of service available at public facilities often leads to "bypassing"—individuals forgo the closest and cheapest public option for health care in favor of higher quality, more distant facilities that carry a much higher cost for treatment than projected in the public system (Filmer et al. 2000). This phenomenon contributes to a situation in which "high catastrophic spending and poverty co-exist with significant economic inequality and poverty in Guatemala" (Bowser and Mahal 2010). A powder keg of uninsured individuals concentrated in rural areas, low levels of access to health care, and overall low levels of insurance coverage means that the slightest ongoing malady or most sudden illness can be "economically devastating" to a household (Bowser and Mahal 2010).

Exceptionally vulnerable segments of society

In sum, a number of issues, including poverty, lack of access, ineffective services, and insufficient government investment have left Guatemala with superlatively negative scores in most major indicators of poverty and public health when compared to other countries in Latin America and the Caribbean. In 2003, Guatemalans had the highest infant mortality in Central America and the lowest life expectancy at 65 years of age (Gragnolati and Marini 2003). More recent reports indicate that as of 2010 life expectancy had increased to seventy-one years, still well below the seventy-eight years expectancy in the United States and seventy-seven years in Mexico (World Bank n.d.b).

Fifty-six percent of Guatemalan families in 2003 were living below the poverty line, and 16 percent lived in extreme poverty, unable to purchase a basic basket of food (Gragnolati and Marini 2003). In fact, Bowser and Mahal (2010) claim that Guatemala is characterized by the greatest total percentage of the population living below the poverty line of all Latin American and Caribbean countries. In 2006, the percentage of the overall population living below the poverty line of $1.25 a day (PPP adjusted) was shockingly high—51 percent—when compared with the average of 8 percent for all Latin American and Caribbean countries. This means that at least half of all Guatemalan families struggle to put even basic foods on the table, let alone nutritious and diverse foods. Consequently, Guatemala has been identified as the most chronically malnourished country in Latin America (44 percent of the population; Gragnolati and Marini 2003).

Indigenous and rural populations

In 2009, *The Economist* described malnutrition in Guatemala as "A National Shame." The country's malnutrition rate was ranked sixth-worst in the world (*The Economist* 2009). For Guatemala's indigenous Maya people, who constitute the majority of rural dwellers, this situation is even bleaker. Disaggregating the data by ethnicity, *The Economist* found:

> In parts of rural Guatemala, where the population is overwhelmingly of Mayan descent, the incidence of child malnutrition reaches 80 percent. A diet of little more than tortillas does permanent damage….
> In Jocotán, in the east, rehabilitation centres have admitted dozens of children who are so malnourished that their black hair has turned blond, their faces are chubby from fluid build-up as their organs fail, the veins in their legs become a visible black spider-web and their face

muscles are too weak to smile. What makes this even more distressing
is that Guatemala is rich enough to prevent it.

Because indigenous and rural populations are consistently underrepre-
sented in the census and aggregated into the general national statistics,
estimates of total health in Guatemala do not accurately represent the
critical state of health for the more than 40 percent of the population that
is Mayan, nor those living in more remote regions of the country (PNUD
2010, Minority Rights Group International 2009).

When disaggregation by ethnicity is possible, health indicators for
the indigenous population in Guatemala appear even more disturbing
than already grim statistics for the country as a whole. Seventy-six percent of the indigenous population lived below the poverty line in 2010,
with 27 percent in extreme poverty. In fact, health outcome indicators
are consistently worse for the indigenous populations, especially in the
areas of infant and child mortality, child morbidity, and use of health services (Beckett and Pebley 2003, Goldman et al. 2000). Child malnutrition
among the indigenous population has improved in the last twenty-five
years, from 71.7 percent in 1987 to 58.6 percent in 2008/2009, though
a significant difference still separates this neglected group from the 30.6
percent child malnutrition rate among the non-indigenous community
(PNUD 2010).

This disparity may be attributed in part to the fact that health
care services are not culturally accessible to Mayan populations, whose
language and belief systems are different from the dominant language
and culture of the ladino population (Goldman et al. 2000). The ladino
population is a discrete ethnic group, "a heterogeneous population which
expresses itself in the Spanish language as a maternal language, which
possesses specific traits of Hispanic origin mixed with indigenous cultural
elements, and dresses in a style commonly considered Western" (Quirós
and Arias 2007). According to official estimates, ladinos constitute half of
the total Guatemalan population. Historically, this group has controlled a
disproportionate amount of political, economic, and sociocultural power
over the country's indigenous groups.

But much more important than cultural difference per se has been
violence; as Levy and Sidel aptly state, "War is anathema to public health.
… As a result of wars, many people have inadequate access to food, clean
water, medical care, and other conditions necessary for public health…
Refugees and internally displaced persons are vulnerable to malnutrition,
infectious diseases, injuries, and criminal military acts" (2003: 167). The
decades of aggression directed at Guatemala's considerable indigenous
population has led to institutionalized discrimination against Maya peo-

ples, whose residence is now concentrated in remote, rural areas that are underserved by public spending (see May 2001, Smith 1990, Carmack 1988). The World Bank also attributes the dire health outcomes of the "indigenous subpopulation" to decades of war, explaining, "several thousand people have been displaced as a result of internal strife. The majority of those who returned to Guatemala resettled in the most remote areas, where they are now living in precarious conditions with limited access to basic services" (Gragnolati and Marini 2003: 2).

Although the indigenous population is disproportionately concentrated in rural areas, all rural people tend to be excluded from most social, educational, and economic opportunities to improve their well-being. The considerable disparity between rich and poor populations in Guatemala is widely recognized by domestic and international bodies alike, leading the WHO to describe health care as a "luxury good" in countries such as Guatemala (Makinen et al. 2000). In such cases, "richer groups tend to spend a higher percentage of their consumption on health care than do poorer groups" and "these wealthier households allocated a higher percentage of their overall consumption spending to health care" (Makinen et al. 2000: 62).

As a result, poorer residents living in rural areas tend to have lower scores in health indicators than do their urban dwelling counterparts. For example, in 1996 child mortality among rural residents was estimated at 74 per 1000 live births, compared to 55 per 1000 in urban areas (Goldman et al. 2001). In 2003, the World Bank described Guatemala as the least urbanized country in Central America, with only 39 percent of the population residing in urban areas (Gragnolati and Marini 2003). Though malnutrition is a nationwide chronic health problem in Guatemala, the rate in rural areas (51.8 percent) is considerably worse than in urban areas (28.8 percent) (PNUD 2010).

The overall poor health conditions of rural and indigenous Guatemalans means that poisoning from agrochemical exposure is difficult for farmers to recognize independently as a serious medical problem. The symptoms of pesticide poisoning include headache, nausea, diarrhea, fatigue, loss of coordination, and confusion (EPA 2012). According to the EPA (2012), these symptoms mimic more benign medical concerns, such as heat exhaustion, common in the context of agricultural labor. Furthermore, the symptoms of pesticide poisoning bear a striking resemblance to two of the most prevalent medical concerns resulting from rural standards of living—acute respiratory infections and diarrhea associated with poor hygienic conditions and unsanitary drinking water (Montgomery and Elimelech 2007, Prüss-Üstün et al. 2004, Evans et al. 2004,

Gragnolati and Marini 2003, Aiello and Larson 2002, Goldman et al. 2001).

Unfortunately, the commonality of illnesses such as diarrhea and acute respiratory infections combined with the lack of access to and prohibitive costs of health care forces families to make difficult decisions on whether or not to seek professional treatment. An investigation of beliefs about illness in four Guatemalan departments documented that only 31 percent of respondents suggested diarrhea might be caused by hygienic conditions, while 26 percent of respondents also cited non-biomedical causes such as hot/cold imbalance, eating too much fruit, or eating at the wrong time of day, none of which necessitate professional medical attention (Goldman et al. 2000). Another study found that severity of symptoms, duration of illness, and especially time missed from work are the most influential factors in families' decisions to seek medical attention (Weller et al. 1997). In the absence of proper training on toxic pesticide exposure or accessible health care, agricultural families living in rural conditions plagued by unsafe drinking water and overwhelming poverty often fail to recognize the signs or gravity of agrochemical poisoning.

Illiterate and undereducated populations

In the literature on factors that contribute to public health, literacy is frequently cited as an important contributor to improved health outcomes (Rudd et al. 2000). Literacy enhances individuals' ability to follow health care and treatment instructions, whereas illiteracy hinders individuals from seeking treatment because they face difficulty and embarrassment in registering for services (Rudd et al. 2000). Literacy also is associated with greater knowledge of health services and care, lower rates of hospitalization, more positive scores on global measures of health, and lower rates of chronic disease (DeWalt et al. 2004). Education in general is associated with disease prevention: more educated individuals tend to adopt more health conscious values and lifestyles, work in safer and healthier environments, and feel more confident in asserting their rights in unsafe working conditions (Rudd et al. 2000).

In Guatemala, literacy rates have steadily improved since 1989, when only 79.6 percent of the urban population (age 15 and over) and 48.2 percent of the rural population were considered literate. Literacy has recently reached 86 percent among the urban population and 62.3 percent among rural Guatemalans (PNUD 2010). Minority Rights Group International disaggregates these figures to demonstrate the indigenous/ ladino disparity in literacy, finding 91 percent of ladino males and 86 percent of urban ladino women are literate, compared with 75 percent of indigenous males and just 55 percent of urban indigenous women (Minority Rights Group International 2009). Looking specifically at the population between 15 and 24 years of age, literacy rates are much higher at 94.5 percent and 81.1 percent in urban and rural areas, respectively (PNUD 2010). At the *básico* level of education (grades six–eight), indigenous students now comprise 22 percent of the school-going population. Because literacy rates among children are higher, it is not uncommon for parents to ask their offspring to read and interpret for them important and official documents.

Illiteracy and insufficient education further endanger agricultural workers by leaving them at higher risk of agrochemical poisoning, as farmers are oftentimes unable to read the instructions on chemical containers that are essential to proper usage. Following international recommendations, pesticide manufacturers have developed a color coding system to symbolically indicate the severity or level of danger presented by a particular product. However, a study by Popper et al. (1996) found these cues inadequate, as they only relate relative levels of danger without effectively conveying the intended use of the product. More broadly, in a study of a Safe Pesticide Use training program, Popper et al. found that farmers who had completed training demonstrated greater reported knowledge of many best practices in chemical application. For example, 78 percent of the farmers surveyed who had completed training could accurately identify the instant of opening the chemical container as the moment in which poisoning is most dangerous. Among farmers who had not received training, only 37 percent of those surveyed provided the same accurate response.

Comparing the actions of participants in the Safe Pesticide Use program with farmers who did not participate, however, the study found that farmers in both groups still practiced inappropriate pesticide application. Both trained and untrained farmers inaccurately stated that application dosages should be based on the number of pests, when in fact dosages should be gauged according to surface area alone. In practice, this means that the vast majority of farmers were treating severe pest infestations with severe applications of agricultural chemicals. Farmers in both groups reported applying pesticides to treat fungus outbreaks in their fields, which not only is ineffective fungus management strategy, but also can have the unintended effect of conditioning existing pests to tolerate higher dosages of chemical application. Vendors may be exacerbating this dilemma as they seek to increase sales by promoting a "more is better" application philosophy in places where farmers have increased access

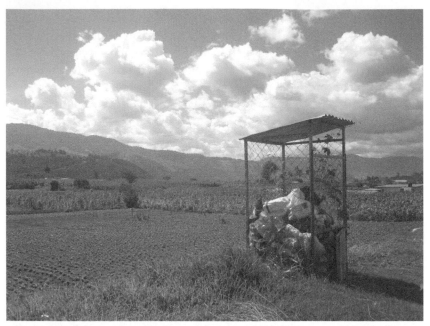

Figure 2.1.   Container for disposal of used chemical packages, including a discarded Antracol fungicide package.

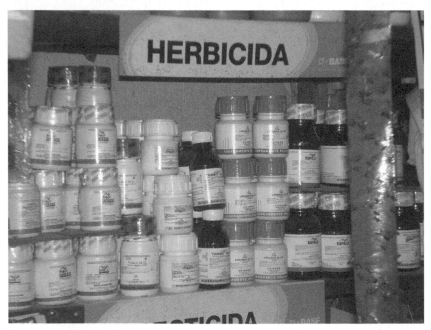

Figure 2.2.   Herbicides of varying toxicity on the shelves of an agrochemical store.

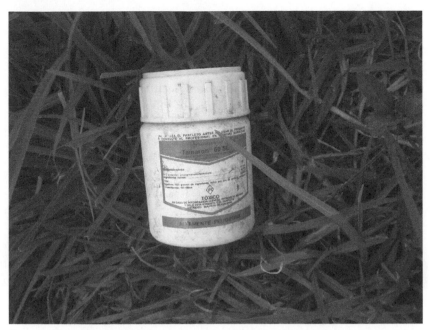

Figure 2.3.   One of several used containers of Tamaron (now a banned insecticide) we found in the fields.

to chemical products but insufficient information about product safety (Corriols Molina 2009, Hogstedt et al 2007, Guidotti and Gitterman 2007, Mull and Kirkhorn 2005, Mathews et al. 2003, Popper et al. 1996).

Farmers overall demonstrated an alarming unfamiliarity with the causes, symptoms, and treatment of agrochemical poisoning. Despite the fact that 64 percent of the chemicals used by farmers in the Popper et al. study fell into the "extremely toxic" category, farmers only identified milder health effects of pesticide poisoning—headaches, nausea, vomiting, and dizziness. Rarely did farmers suggest more severe consequences such as cancer and birth defects. Similarly, when asked how poisoning occurs, farmers in the study most often described an incidence of ingestion and rarely mentioned skin contact, which is the most common avenue for exposure poisoning. Finally, the study found very little knowledge among farmers of effective manners of treatment of poisoned individuals. Only 30 percent offered adequate reactions to poisoning, such as washing and inducing vomiting. More commonly, farmers simply did not know of a treatment or suggested such colloquial and dangerously inaccurate remedies as lemonade and black coffee.

Women and children among the laboring population

The numerous factors negatively affecting public health in Guatemala—poverty, illiteracy, discrimination, malnutrition, corruption—also enhance the danger of toxic agrochemical use in agriculture. For example, poverty drives women and children to join the labor force in order to supplement their household income (London et al. 2002). However, women and children often comprise an invisible working class. They may work in their family fields or accompany men who work as paid agricultural laborers, where the participation of women and children is typically unauthorized. Children often work during vacations and seasonal breaks from school. In fact, according to the World Bank, one in eight children in the developing world is engaged in child labor, and among laboring children, seven in ten work in agriculture (Fares and Raju 2007).

The historically lesser social status of women in Guatemala combined with a number of other social and cultural conditions render women and children among the most vulnerable populations at risk of pesticide poisoning (Calvert et al. 2003). Both women and children are generally less experienced as employees laboring under a supervisor. Therefore they are likely to lack the confidence, or the authorization, to question their assigned duties or assert their rights to a safe working environment (Calvert et al. 2003). They are more likely to be engaged as seasonal or temporary workers, tenuous positions that receive less investment in their long-term well-being, safety training, or equipment (Mull and Kirkhorn 2005, Calvert et al. 2003, London et al. 2002).

As informal and elusive members of the working class, women and children tend to be underestimated as laborers affected by agrochemical poisoning and their exposure to pesticides is notoriously difficult to measure (London et al. 2002, Panjabi 2010, Fares and Raju 2007). A study of cocoa growers in Ghana found that children had little knowledge of proper chemical handling even though they were assigned such hazardous tasks as mixing, loading sprayers, and applying chemicals (Mull and Kirkhorn 2005). They work with such inadequate protection as open-toed shoes, shorts, and sleeveless shirts. Children involved in cotton cultivation in India reported frequent headaches, dizziness, and skin and eye irritations after spraying pesticides without proper safety equipment or water to wash exposed areas.

We know that toxic chemical exposure is especially damaging to children. In the agricultural sector in the developing world, employed children demonstrate more negative health outcome indicators—including higher mortality and morbidity, higher malnutrition, and lower school

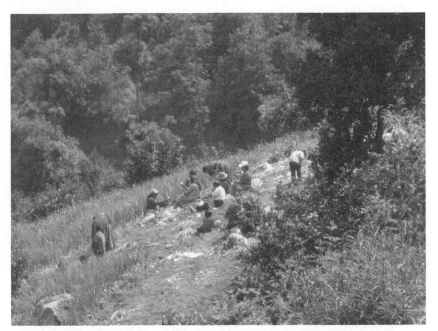

Figure 2.4.   A working crew primarily composed of women and children pulling onions on a hillside.

enrollment rates—than their unemployed counterparts (Panjabi 2010). Because their physical bodies are still in formative stages, and their systems function on a smaller scale, pesticides become more concentrated in children's systems and the effects of poisoning are exaggerated and longer-term (Calvert et al. 2003, Harari et al. 1997). For example, a 1997 study of exposure to toxic chemicals among child laborers in Ecuador identified elevated levels of numerous industrial compounds including pesticides, benzene, lead, and mercury in children's urine samples. Highlighting the specific risks of these chemicals to exposed child workers, the study noted that many such chemicals are rarely found in samples given by workers in developed countries or among adult workers in general (Harari et al. 1997).

The tasks that women and children are typically assigned in agricultural work are intended to capitalize on their supposed advantages in manual dexterity. As a result, they typically are responsible for harvesting activities that involve extensive manual contact with planted crops, usually shortly after a pesticide treatment (Mull and Kirkhorn 2005, London et al. 2002, Harari et al. 1997). These harvesting activities should be conducted with hand protection to prevent direct contact with pesticides and minimize cuts and skin abrasions that create open conduits for pesticides to enter the blood stream. In the majority of cases, these workers do not have access to protective equipment when working.

Women face a number of other opportunities for pesticide poisoning that are typically overlooked or unanticipated by public health workers. A study examining women's exposure to agriculture chemicals in developing countries found that, though their exposure is consistently underestimated and unreported, their non-occupational opportunities for chemical exposure exceed those of male agricultural workers due to the typical division of labor in a developing country such as Guatemala (London et al. 2002). For example, mothers and daughters typically wash the clothing of men in the household, leaving women to handle the chemical-coated pants and long-sleeved shirts they carry to the washbasin. In many cases, women also engage in paid labor as washerwomen in their communities, magnifying their opportunities for chemical exposure. Women often remain indoors for the majority of the day, as many do in Guatemala, and when toxic pesticides have been sprayed indoors to kill pests such as fleas and cockroaches, they are constantly exposed to fumes as they conduct their daily chores.

In fact, the safety of the entire household is in jeopardy where pesticides are included in growing practices, but training for responsible handling is inadequate, particularly where women are excluded from training programs altogether. London et al. (2002) provide ample scenarios in which agrochemicals are reintroduced into the home, such as reuse of chemical containers for food storage, storage of chemicals in the kitchen near the food supply, and providing contaminated feed to livestock. Similarly, Popper et al.'s 1996 study of the impacts of Safe Pesticide Use training found that, despite gains in training men on responsible handling, women reported applying pesticides to treat insects in the home, such as mosquitoes, fleas, and even head lice. According to the researchers, women not included in the Safe Pesticide Use program did not differentiate between pests in the field and pests in the home; they presumed the same treatment to be effective for both. Evidently, even when safety equipment and proper training is provided for chemical handling in the field, the dangers of pesticides extend outside the field and into the home, particularly along channels of typical women's work in developing countries.

Beyond regulation: socioeconomic factors that enhance public health risks

Despite the best efforts of the international community and farmers themselves to make agricultural production safer, in Guatemala, as in many countries of the developing world, a complex set of issues allows dangerous agrochemical use to persist. These issues are layered one upon another, so that global processes (such as expanding avenues of trade) impact the choices of national leaders (for example, to remove protections for worker safety), which in turn affect the actions of producers, who exploit themselves and their family's labor in order to maintain a competitive edge in the global market. As a result, the educational efforts and trade policies designed to foster best practices in safe handling of chemicals are inherently inadequate, as they can only address isolated aspects of dangerous agrochemical application. These regulations have been unable to encompass all the problems of poor health care systems, lack of education, malnutrition, and economically desperate populations that are so common among agriculture laborers in developing countries such as Guatemala.

The structural and infrastructural characteristics of life in developing countries not only undermine attempts to make agriculture safer, but also serve to render agricultural laborers particularly vulnerable to the dangers of agrochemical use. While the expansion of the global market provides greater opportunities for farmers to earn a profit, the freer circulation of goods also means that unregulated and banned chemicals reach populations that are especially ill prepared to make sound judgments about chemical use. At the same time that poverty drives agricultural laborers to take risks in production, it also excludes them from resources such as education and health care that would provide a safety net to counterbalance these risks.

As apparent as the risks of agrochemical application seem, and as high as the long-term costs of agrochemical dependency are, it is difficult to understand why farmers would willingly continue to jeopardize the safety of their families and their communities. But for farmers it is less a deliberate choice and more an unstoppable momentum that drives them to defy so many warnings. Economic necessity, lack of alternatives, and the pressing needs created by the global economy—to remain competitive, to independently cover health costs, to earn enough to match rising costs of living—keep many farmers locked into a series of interrelated, hazardous practices that are increasingly difficult to escape.

In the next chapter, we provide a glimpse into the lives of coffee growers to see how global, national, and personal factors combine to turn a seemingly easy choice—to break the cycle of chemical application and switch to organic production techniques—into an unbelievably difficult decision.

Chapter 3

A Community Torn:
Struggling to Rectify Agrochemical Hazards and the Immediate Needs Treadmill

The winds of 2007 have become the stuff of legend in Bella Vista. In March of that year, the coffee plants had just begun to flower, dotting the mountainsides with tufts of white blossoms. It was the season for clearing shade trees so that the sun could beam down and fortify the blooms that would soon turn to fruits. For families who were enjoying success in their organic production techniques, the prospects looked good that this harvest would be even better than the last. For families who had not seen such favorable results from organic conversion, this year would drive them deeper into conventional production and push them even further away from abandoning agrochemicals.

Without warning, a vicious storm tore through the community, first whipping the coffee trees with violent winds. Then, unseasonably torrential downpours that lasted for three days washed away the fallen blossoms. Residents of Bella Vista have not forgotten the devastation that was the 2007–2008 harvest. Coffee trees were stripped bare, leaving nothing behind to catch the sun, nothing to transform into coffee cherry, nothing to pick, and nothing to sell. Coffee production tends to be cyclical, alternating good years and bad years. But production volumes for that year were less than half the quantity of a bad year. Bills still had to be paid, costs had to be recouped, emergencies still arose though there were no household funds to cover them, and the farmers scrambled to survive another year until the next chance for their annual income rolled around.

The residents who have persisted with organic techniques responded to the winds of 2007 by relying on their umbrella cooperative. They negotiated with their foreign buyer for subsidized profits for the little harvest they could scrape together. They worked extra hours in construction, clearing land, picking coffee on other plantations, or wherever possible to cover their losses. And they planted more trees, ripping up the old and now battered coffee plants and replacing them with new seedlings. But

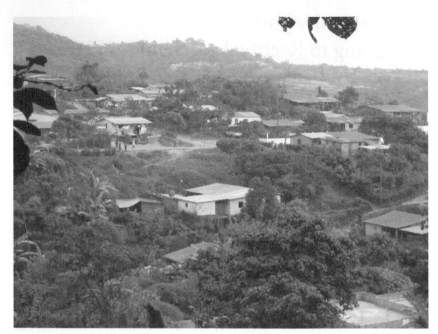

Figure 3.1.   The community of Bella Vista, viewed from a coffee plot.

the residents who had reverted back to conventional techniques sold their meager harvest in the local market, collecting what profits they could to pay off debts at home. Unable to invest in the costs or labor needed for new plants, they spent as much as they could manage on the chemical fertilizer urea, hoping to kick-start production into overdrive for the subsequent harvest, still a year away.

The disparate responses of the two groups in the community to the disaster of the 2007 winds reflect the challenge of the more persistent dilemma they face: how to work toward the future when the present is so unbearably demanding. This chapter follows the stories of Don Efraín and Doña Marcelina to see how conversion to organic production requires taking serious risks and waiting patiently for results. But not all coffee growers are equally prepared to bear the short-term costs of organic conversion. For farmers in a more precarious situation, agrochemicals are associated with safety and security and predictable success. Though all residents of Bella Vista are undoubtedly committed to the long-term health of the community, household needs understandably take precedence. In this chapter, we investigate the many factors that mount to trap coffee growers on a treadmill of immediate needs; we also explore the resources that allow some farmers to escape.

One community, two cooperatives

Tucked away on the steep slope of the Santa Maria Volcano, the community of Bella Vista is currently home to about 145 families, over 1000 residents. The community was established in the mid-1970s when the Catholic Church purchased the land as a refuge for ten *finca* (plantation) workers and their families. A Spanish priest had been working in the rural countryside of Guatemala, clandestinely training indigenous finca workers to become catechists, though their bosses would not grant them the liberty to attend public events such as religious services. For years, several finca workers pleaded with the priest for help to escape the exploitative life of the finca. After a near-decade of petitioning the international Catholic community, the priest eventually acquired the funds to buy the workers a finca of their own. The finca he purchased was placed in the name of the Bella Vista farmer cooperative. Each resident was granted usage rights, rather than ownership, to designated plots of land. Today, the overwhelming majority of residents continue to participate in the cooperative, cultivating coffee in their plots, turning in their product to the community processing facility, and eventually receiving payment for their contribution.

As they left behind their lives as plantation workers, the heads of the ten founding families of Bella Vista brought to the cooperative considerable knowledge and experience in conventional cultivation methods. Consequently, they began coffee production in Bella Vista using the only techniques they knew. For more than twenty years, the cooperative sold conventionally produced coffee, monitoring prices and negotiating their own trade agreements with purchasers in Guatemala's major trading and processing hubs of Escuintla and Coatepeque. But in 2000, a series of events, both global and local, culminated in the decision to pursue organic certification and sell coffee through fair trade channels.

Organic and fair trade are two distinct forms of coffee certification, wherein producers meet a series of requirements in order to receive a "premium" price. Cooperatives are increasingly dual-certified because fair trade producers are pressured to pursue organic certification (Calo and Wise 2005); about 80% of fair trade certified coffee sold in the United States is also organic certified (Raynolds 2002). According to Lyon (2009: 224), "the organic coffee market attempts to bridge the geographic and cultural differences between consumers and producers by forging relations of solidarity rooted in economic justice and environmental stewardship." Despite consumer sentiments of solidarity, coffee growers usually associate organic certification with requirements that guarantee the material quality of the coffee, such as absence of chemical residues and exceptional grade beans, while fair trade certification speaks more to the symbolic quality, such as the social terms of trade (Bray et al. 2002, Bacon 2005, Jaffee 2007).

A global coffee glut accompanied by commodity price speculation saw international coffee prices vary wildly throughout the 1990s and early 2000s, ranging from $.40 per pound in 1992 to $1.02 per pound in 1998. Following this peak, the price slid again, dropping to $.70 per pound by 2000. This is when Bella Vista first obtained organic and fair trade certification (ICO n.d. a, ICO n.d. b).

The decision to convert from conventional production was introduced by the Spanish priest who succeeded the cooperative's original benefactor (who had been forced to leave Guatemala during the civil violence of the 1980s to mid-1990s). The new priest promoted organic cultivation as a means of securing a better coffee price in the fixed-price fair trade system and developing more environmentally responsible growing practices, thereby protecting the natural resources of the mountainside community. The residents of Bella Vista received training and materials to make the conversion to organic production from the local umbrella cooperative, Toro Verde. In converting to organic production and joining Toro Verde, the Bella Vista cooperative joined a network of other coffee cooperatives in Guatemala who work together to achieve economies of scale in filling contracts and paying fees. Toro Verde has helped them negotiate new contracts with foreign purchasers and navigate the logistics of selling organic and fair trade certified coffee to the foreign market.

For seven years, the residents of Bella Vista continued to produce and sell as a unified cooperative with organic and fair trade certification. Residents learned to use new organic cultivation techniques, centering on use of organic fertilizer rather than the standard urea, manual weed control rather than use of herbicide, and integrated pest management rather than application of pesticides. To the residents of Bella Vista, the change in cultivation techniques presented a number of tradeoffs, and some families adapted to the change more readily than others.

Organic fertilizer, for example, proved the most contentious feature of organic production. To its credit, the cost of materials to create organic fertilizer is considerably lower than the price of chemical fertilizer. In its most complex form, organic fertilizer is a mixture comprised of brush, yeast, ash, molasses or *panela* (brown sugar cake), and either chicken excrement or cattle manure. Most residents independently produce some variation of fertilizer in-house, using kitchen scraps, coffee pulp, brush, tree trimmings, and ash from the hearth. Also available for purchase in the community is vermicompost, produced in the community's vermiculture project, where red wriggler worms convert coffee pulp, a by-product of coffee production, into nutrient-rich fertilizer. Organic fertilizer can also be purchased outside the community, at prices ranging from US$2.56–3.84 (20–30 GTQ) per *quintal* or 100-pound sack.

Application of organic fertilizer, however, requires a substantially greater investment of time and effort than does its chemical counterpart. One 100-pound sack of organic fertilizer is sufficient to cover only a half-*cuerda* (1 *cuerda* = 43.7 m^2) of coffee plants. The average coffee grower in Bella Vista cultivates 15 cuerdas of coffee, so that full application on all one's cultivated land would require 30 quintales, or 3000 pounds of organic fertilizer. Moreover, coffee plots in Bella Vista are spread throughout the hillsides, with each family responsible for one plot near the village and a second at a more remote location. On average, the closest plots are situated a 20-minute walk away from the village. Following organic cultivation techniques, then, coffee growers carry these 100-pound sacks for a minimum of 20 minutes per trip to reach their nearest plots, and the trip must be repeated about 30 times each year.

Chemical fertilizer offers ease of application, though at a higher financial cost. One quintal of urea, purchased at an agrochemical store outside the community, costs around US$38.46 (300 GTQ) and covers about three cuerdas of coffee plants. To cover all cultivated land, the average coffee grower in Bella Vista would need to purchase five quintales of urea, at a cost of around US$192.31 (1500 GTQ), compared to US$115.38 (900 GTQ) to cover one's entire cultivated area using organic fertilizer. There is, however, a clear advantage in hauling five, rather than thirty, quintales of fertilizer to a coffee plot located twenty minutes away.

After the first few years of organic production, unrest began brewing within the cooperative. Some farmers struggled to comply with organic certification requirements. Some complained that organic best practices had damaged their coffee plants. Others still balked that the price was not high enough to compensate for the additional work. As a result, a few families reverted back to chemical fertilizers. Gradually these families drew the support of more residents to return to conventional production. After repeated demands for a community vote, an election was held in 2006 to determine the fate of coffee production in Bella Vista: Would they continue as an organic certified cooperative? Or would they resume conventional coffee production?

The vote resulted in a near tie; fifty-two families opted to continue organic cultivation and fifty-one families chose to convert back to conventional methods. Rather than insist that one group assume the cultivation techniques of the other, the community decided to split the cooperative into two groups. The Organic Group would continue working with Toro Verde to sell organic and fair trade certified coffee, though with half the cooperative's size and, therefore, half the production volume available to fill contracts. The Conventional Group would discontinue organic practices and resume selling to their former buyer in the conventional coffee market.

We now consider two cases—Don Efraín, leader of the Conventional Group, and Doña Marcelina, daughter of one of the founding members of the community—to understand what it means to be an organic or conventional producer, the challenges posed by organic production, and the solutions to these challenges that Organic Group members have found through participation in the Toro Verde cooperative.

We are paying for it now:
Don Efraín and the Conventional Group

Waking well before sunrise, Don Efraín washes his face at the wash basin just outside as Doña Zenaida prepares the day's fire in the kitchen stove. The firewood now transformed into a pile of glowing hot embers, Doña Zenaida gingerly flips tortillas on the scorching hot griddle using the tips of her fingers. She boils a pot of water for coffee and scrambles eggs in a skillet for Don Efraín's breakfast. As he packs his meal to-go, he grabs an extra bottle of sugared water and sets out across the creek, zigzagging uphill through the date palm, following the ridge separating Bella Vista from the neighboring estate, until he reaches his coffee plots thirty-five minutes later.

After two hours of laborious weeding, bent at the waist, swinging a machete just inches above the ground to clear away the ever-present brush, Don Efraín sits for a morning break in the shade. Ignoring the mosquitoes and biting gnats swarming around his face, he pries open the plastic tubs containing a stack of tortillas and some eggs with sliced hot dogs. As Don Efraín regards the coffee plants surrounding him, he admires all the green cherries dotting the branches. Though the newest additions to his plot were only two years old, already they had matured enough to contribute a little to the annual harvest. After several years of disastrously low production, Don Efraín felt he was finally getting back on track. This year would be a good year.

After finishing his breakfast, Don Efraín returns to work, grabbing branches high overhead and trimming away the shade canopy that trapped moisture, caused fungal outbreaks, and prevented sunlight from warming his plants. He gathers all the trimmings into a pile at the back of his plot, leaving them to decay and transform into the compost that would eventually fertilize his new plants. After the sun passes overhead and begins its slow descent, Don Efraín packs his lunch containers and thermos in his backpack, slides his machete back into its holder on his hip, and heads back down the mountainside. Though he reaches home exhausted and drenched in sweat, an instant in the ice cold shower revives him for the school council meeting, to be followed by a choir practice at the church, and finally concludes the evening with a meeting of the Conventional Group to discuss when to open the coffee processing facility for the season, all before Doña Zenaida has the dinner tortillas on the table.

A pillar of the community, Don Efraín has held offices in most of its major decision-making bodies. Due to his respected status as an active catechist in Bella Vista, as well as his diplomacy in communicating with the Organic Group, Don Efraín has been repeatedly nominated as leader of the Conventional Group. He is a reluctant leader, however, expressing more concern than support for the use of chemicals in coffee production. To talk to Don Efraín about agrochemicals, one would guess that he is a member of the Organic Group.

> For example, in conventional, what they use is poison. To fumigate. But this is dangerous for your health. You have to use a mask. And carry it in a backpack and fumigate like this [gestures a spraying action] on the leaves. But it is poison. They will see it in an analysis. It can kill a person. So, it works for sicknesses, for disease [in coffee plants]. However, we do not buy this because it scares us. It scares us for our health.

Like most all residents in Bella Vista, Don Efraín tried organic production techniques for several years. Like most members of the Conventional Group, Don Efraín believes that organic certification was far more work than the compensation that organic prices offered during the years 2000–2007. He, and others like him, felt foolish hauling 100-pound sacks uphill for a 35-minute walk, scouring coastal cities for organic seedlings, and painstakingly inspecting each individual coffee cherry, only to receive a negligibly better price than farmers in the next village over, who bought seedlings wherever the prices were best and simply sprinkled a little urea on their plants.

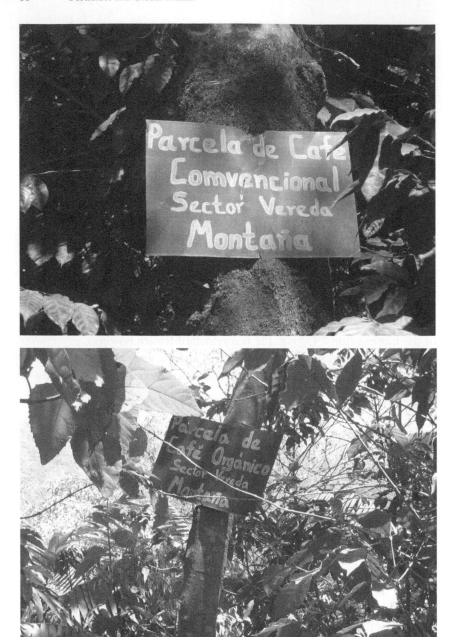

Figures 3.2 and 3.3.   Hand painted signs distinguish between conventional (top) and organic (bottom) coffee plots.

Don Efraín's plots are now demarcated with *cola de gallo*, a native plant with slender, reddish-purple leaves that resemble the plumes of a rooster tail. Not only do they provide a visible barrier distinguishing his from the surrounding plots, but the roots of the plant grow deep and hungry enough that they construct a physical barrier between Don Efraín's conventional plots and the plots of a neighbor in the Organic Group. Included in the two-cooperative arrangement was the pledge by the Conventional Group to respect the decision of Organic Group members and make every effort to contain their chemical use. The *cola de gallo* serves to protect organic plots from any chemicals that could leach into the soil. Furthermore, Conventional Group members must abstain from any chemical application that could jeopardize the Organic Group's certified status. As a result, the conventional group is still prohibited from using pesticides, fungicides, or herbicides in the coffee plots. Most residents are willing to abide by this rule, though some in the Conventional Group have sneaked herbicide applications, prompting rebuke from cooperative leaders and threats of a hefty fine if the practice continued.

With the exception of a few unauthorized herbicides, most members of the Conventional Group see a qualitative difference in fertilizers, pesticides, herbicides, and fungicides. Don Efraín recognizes the negative effects of chemical weed killers on the land. "You are not going to spray Gramoxone, they [Organic Group] said. You are not going to apply Gramoxone because if you do you will wash out the land. The land will wash away when it rains. So, by machete, just with a machete, we weed the *cafetal* (coffee plot)." The residents of Bella Vista have deep appreciation for their natural resources, and they recognize the damage that chemical use has inflicted upon the environment in the lower-elevation coffee regions nearby.

> If we apply more fertilizers, chemicals, or poisons it causes more contamination of the environment. And the air carries it and one breathes it, right? The air is no longer pure. It is air contaminated with poison. Yes. On the other hand, here the environment is pure, because there is more organic [coffee] that does not use chemical. It is not conventional. So you breathe pure air. Notice when you go down there to the coast, you can sense the unpleasant odors. ... You do not breathe well there. There are some ugly odors. On the other hand, here, no. So that is why we also do not use much. Because chemicals, for example, in the fumigation of plants you notice a smell like pure garlic. Although garlic is food. It is good for health. But this is poison. It goes for analysis, and it affects the lungs.

According to the manufacturer of Gramoxone, the active ingredient Paraquat "does not have a negative effect on ground water or soil organisms, even after five years of repeated applications." Gramoxone is "still one of the most widely used herbicides in the world." According to the Pesticide Action Network, the dangers of Graxomone extend beyond Efraín's environmental concerns. In fact, PAN asserts that dermal contact with Paraquat can cause fissures, loss of fingernails, and ulceration. Inhalation symptoms appear as a cough, headache, sore throat, or labored breathing (Kegley et al. 2010). Paraquat is highly toxic when ingested and has been associated with a number of accidental poisonings and an even higher number of suicides (see also Kolilekas et al. 2006; Fernando et al. 1990; Parkinson 1980). Poisoning ultimately resulting in fatal pulmonary fibrosis, which may take several days to manifest and can be worsened by physical exertion.

While Don Efraín has found acceptable replacements for pesticide, fungicide, and herbicide, he has not had success with organic production techniques. The chemical fertilizer urea, on the other hand, is seen by Don Efraín and others in the Conventional Group as an essential component of coffee production. Residents speak of urea application in maternal terms; as a mother cares for her children, so do they give coffee plants the necessary nutrients for their healthy development. In contrast, stories abound within the Conventional Group relating the disaster of organic cultivation practices, particularly the method of digging a half-moon trench around the roots to encourage root growth. Several members of the Conventional Group found organic cultivation techniques to be harmful to the health of their coffee plots. Rather than boost production as intended, Don Efraín found the half-moon fertilizing technique instead damaged his plants: "They wanted us to make trenches around the base, supposedly for the good of the coffee. ... And in our harvest? Year after year, year after year, years passed and we did not grow anything. Today we are still [restoring] our coffee plots. ... I want to get it back to how it was before. We are paying for it now, and how."

In light of his failed organic experiments, Don Efraín takes a nuanced and cautious view of fertilizer application. Recognizing that chemicals are harmful to human health, he still believes that fertilizers such as urea are vital to the health of coffee plants. Consequently, he and many others in the Conventional Group tend to approach chemical application with an aim to apply as minimally as possible.

> We help them a little. Yes. So that we do not cause much contamination... In the air it takes care of sickness in the plants, but harms us,

the people. I am already seeing sickness in our health. Therefore it is not very good to use poison on the plants. Not much. So for us it is also better to use *cal* (slaked lime used to disinfect the ground before planting), nothing more. Cal we add to the new plants. That is how to kill a little of the sickness.

Adding to the frustration of Don Efraín and other coffee growers in the Conventional Group is the delayed payment schedule intrinsic to the organic system. Though coffee may be shipped for export in December or January, profits typically reach the growers several months after the coffee has arrived at its destination, passed its final inspection, and the payment has been deposited into the bank account of the cooperative. The residents of Bella Vista can spend months sending frantic emails and compulsively checking their account before the payment finally arrives as many as six months later. In the conventional system, on the other hand, growers receive payment almost immediately. Conventional Group members collect their coffee, monitor coffee prices, determine when to sell, and negotiate with their buyer. As they explain, a major benefit of membership in the Conventional Group is that they sell their coffee and receive their payment shortly afterwards.

To other members in the community, and certainly in the eyes of U.S.-based proponents, the payment schedule for organic and fair trade coffee is seen as a benefit of the system. In the design of the organic and fair trade systems, delayed payment is thought to help producers by spreading their income over the course of the year rather than a single influx of cash at harvest season. The delayed payment system often includes a prefinancing option wherein growers can apply for loans on upcoming coffee sales and repay through deductions from their final coffee profits. This arrangement is viewed by some as an advantage of the organic system, as it provides growers access to a source of funding throughout the year, which they can invest in costs of production, such as labor, fertilizer, and new plants. However, the funds are restricted for use in cultivation-related expenses only, and the delay between the moment of sale and the arrival of payment is unbearable for others whose household needs demand swift delivery of funds.

In Don Efraín's household, for example, pressing expenses such as illness do not wait for coffee plants to rebound or for repeated inspections, transport, and evaluations. Don Efraín's only son migrated north almost two years ago to work in construction in the United States, leaving his wife and their four children to live with his father. Not only has this left Don Efraín alone to maintain his coffee plots, as his three married daughters are now dedicated to working the plots of their new families, but the youngest of Don Efraín's grandchildren, just sixteen months old, contracted an upper respiratory infection in infancy, necessitating frequent doctor's visits and expensive prescription medication. Don Efraín's family spends around US$25.58 (200 GTQ) per week in transport alone, ferrying the infant to the clinic in the nearest city of Retalhuleu, not to mention the cost of the doctor's visit and the endless medications they have tried without significant results.

This issue was a major struggle during Efraín's previous time with the organic cooperative. With the urgent financial need to care for an afflicted child, in the absence of family members to assist him in labor-intensive organic production, and with the disappointing price return for organic certified coffee, he struggled to make organic techniques productive and lucrative. In the end, however, he felt he had to take action to support his family, and so Don Efraín resumed applying chemical fertilizer in hopes for a quick recovery of his coffee plants.

Though he applies much less chemical fertilizer than is recommended for effective dosage, and though he does not apply urea to all his plants, organic certification mandates a three-year chemical-free transition period before coffee can be considered organic. As a result, Don Efraín is not likely to rejoin the Organic Group. Some residents who initially joined the Conventional Group have since switched back to organic techniques, but these farmers did not apply chemical fertilizer during their time as conventional growers, primarily due to financial constraints. Don Efraín, however, and many others like him, applied chemical fertilizer in a state of financial panic, in reaction to unsuccessful organic techniques, an exceptionally bad 2007–2008 harvest, and overwhelming health care expenses.

The economic barriers to organic production have only mounted as Don Efraín's medical bills continue to accumulate, the coffee plants demand more intensive application of urea, and the costs of production are hardly covered by profits from the annual sale. Torn between what is best for his family and what is best for the natural resources in his community, Don Efraín chose to opt for the more immediate need of providing for his family in the only way that has proven successful for him—using chemical fertilizers. In his reckoning, to convert back to the organic production techniques that were so burdensome before would be financial self-sabotage. Though he recognizes the health hazards that fertilizers, pesticides, fungicides, and herbicides present to human health, Don Efraín sees conventional cultivation as the only option that will sustain his production volume and produce the profits he needs to support his escalating household expenses.

The members of the Conventional Group, roughly half of the Bella Vista community, sympathize with Don Efraín's struggle. Though urea is the only chemical permitted by Bella Vista's governing body, several instances of clandestine herbicide application indicate the desperation with which coffee growers are grasping at any means available to improve production, even in full knowledge of their devastating effects on environmental and human health.

It is hard work, but it's worth it:
Doña Marcelina and the Organic Group

Hours before dawn, Doña Marcelina builds the day's fire in the stove inside her kitchen. Much like Efrain's wife, she reheats last night's beans, boils a pot of water for sugared coffee, and nimbly flips tortillas with the lightest swipe of her fingers. Meanwhile, two nieces, both of whom have husbands working in the United States, help her wrangle the gang of children under her care, some her own along with the children of neighbors and relatives. Once everyone is fed and packed for the day, the young ones leave for school and the older ones leave for the coffee plots. Despite the more than 90-degree Fahrenheit steamy jungle heat, they each button up a long sleeved shirt and tie an old t-shirt around their faces to serve as protection from the swarms of aggressive mosquitoes.

After about a fifteen-minute walk down the long road winding out of town, Doña Marcelina takes a sharp turn into the woods, leading her family's crew of young men and women to her father's coffee plots. This day they planned to help Don Manuel pick the considerable coffee harvest ripening on the trees. When Don Manuel notices two of the young men moving along the rows of coffee plants at an improbable pace he eyes them suspiciously. After watching them for just a few moments he sees, just as he had suspected, that his grandsons have been stripping branches by the handful, grabbing each and every bean indiscriminately, without regard for color or ripeness. Don Manuel hollers for the boys to stop and join him in his row. In a firm scolding and retraining, he explains to the boys that, though their previous method allowed them to cover double the area, it was a tremendous waste of the coffee harvest. By picking the unripe cherries, they produced an unnecessarily great quantity of green coffee, which would be sold at dramatically lower prices than the high quality coffee picked as ripe, red cherries. Moreover, their coarse handling of the coffee trees, grabbing rather than plucking coffee cherries, could damage the cherry stem, jeopardizing the robustness of next year's harvest.

After filling three 100-pound sacks with coffee, the crew pauses for their breakfasts, pulling up a log or sitting on a yet-empty sack, and prying open their containers filled with scrambled eggs, last night's beans, and atol de maíz, a thick and sweet corn drink. Doña Marcelina glances around at her father's coffee plots, marveling at the abundance of red among the glossy green leaves. One could never guess by appearance alone that her father cultivated one of the oldest plots of coffee in the community. Over the last ten years, he had invested heavily in replacing the old plants, some of them upwards of thirty years old, ages truly unknown, since they were already present upon the settlement of the community. After a decade of hard work, Don Manuel's coffee plants had transformed from one of the most ancient and tired plots to one of the youngest and most productive in Bella Vista—all using only organic techniques.

Doña Marcelina recognizes the short-term advantages held by Conventional Group members. True, the front-end investment of time and effort to establish plants in an organic system of cultivation can seem overbearing. But she recognizes that the gains in conventional methods are all short term. For example, urea requires quarterly reapplication and becomes less effective over time. Farmers using chemical fertilizers must at the very least maintain chemical application year after year for their plants to continue producing the same volume of coffee. Organic fertilizer, on the other hand, demands a hefty upfront investment of time and labor; however, the results last for two years.

This is just one of the many reasons why Doña Marcelina did not hesitate in her vote to maintain organic production. She made the conversion by collaborating with her entire family to transition the coffee plants on all their plots from conventional to organic. Her oldest brother and sister, both teachers outside the community, dedicated every weekend to entire days of working in the coffee plots in order to accomplish this sweeping renovation project. They continue to rotate among her brothers' and sister's plots, working as a team to haul fertilizer and collect coffee cherries.

As a result, the coffee plants of Don Manuel stand as flourishing testament to the efficacy of organic cultivation. To the critics who discredit the half-moon fertilizing technique and argue that coffee plants require chemical fertilizer, Don Manuel emphasizes the distinction between organic and natural production. Natural production refers to the growth of coffee seeds that have been casually tossed on the ground and taken root of their own volition. Don Manuel believes that many in the

Conventional Group were traumatized by what they believe to be an organic production experience because they instead practiced natural production, failing to commit any significant intervention in the growth of the plant. The half-moon technique, for example, is only effective when accompanied by sufficient organic fertilizer application. Unfortunately, some farmers invested only the first day in the field when the half-moon was cut, failing to return for follow-up fertilizer application. As a result, many members of the Conventional Group witnessed the demise of their coffee plants, whose freshly cut roots stretched to tap into new fertilizer and reached nothing but gaping, crescent-shaped trenches. Don Manuel's plants, on the other hand, nourished by the infusion of nutrient-rich organic fertilizer, appear to have increased in production volume and strengthened their roots.

Not only do Organic Group members sing the praises of their new cultivation techniques, they also speak favorably of the auxiliary benefits of organic certification. For example, torrential downpours and gusting winds in 2007 mercilessly injured the plants of every household in Bella Vista, including that of Don Manuel. In a good year, delicate white coffee flowers dot the mountainside during the months of January, February, and March as portents of the coffee cherries to come. However the winds of 2007 effectively whisked away the fruit-producing mechanism of the coffee plants, so that when the harvest months of October and November arrived, it was clear the coffee had been severely damaged by extreme wind and rain early in the growing season.

One crucial difference, however, in the financial impact of the winds, was that members of the Organic Group were aided by their umbrella cooperative, Toro Verde. Thanks to the advocacy of Toro Verde, Bella Vista's buyer agreed to honor his contract terms, regardless of the production volume, by purchasing whatever scant amount of the harvest could be scraped together and paying the original favorable price. A more detached buyer in the conventional market, on the other hand, would likely reject Bella Vista's negligible harvest on the grounds of their failure to deliver the contracted amount of coffee. For such a trivial volume of coffee that the growers in Bella Vista produced that year, processing fees and paperwork may create more work for purchasers than the profits they stand to gain, leaving producers to negotiate a desperate deal with an unknown buyer. Toro Verde, on the other hand, not only pressured the buyer to uphold his terms of trade, but also secured a slight per-pound price increase to help compensate for meager returns on such low production volume.

In fact, according to Doña Marcelina, collaboration and support from Toro Verde is the single biggest benefit of the organic system. For example,

since the coffee growers of Bella Vista knew no other method of cultivation than the conventional techniques they learned on the fincas where
they once lived, they required significant training to convert to organic production. In recognition of this obstacle, Toro Verde offered initial training
courses in organic cultivation techniques, biological pest control, organic
fertilizer production, even accounting. In addition, Toro Verde has provided
financial support for cooperative leaders who wish to specialize in some
stage of production, such as fertilizer production, coffee processing, and
professional coffee tasting (*cupping*). Many members of the Organic Group
view these ongoing workshops as a satisfying form of professional development and an opportunity for adult education that was never possible during
their days on the finca. As Don Manuel explained:

> They brought workshops for the directors, for members, technical
> assistance, and in the last two years, workshops for coffee tasting. They
> have helped us to make a nursery, make an organic fertilizer facility,
> *bokashi*, and because we have continued in this project, now the money
> is coming in to pay for our first kilo of organic fertilizer. Now there is
> a lot… I wanted to get really involved because you learn a lot. Yes, you
> learn a lot. My neighbors say they will not lose their day to someone
> who doesn't pay, but… training here, receiving workshops here, that
> helps us work together as a group.

Elected members of the Organic Group receive additional training to
become *promotores* who patrol coffee plots and offer advice and technical
assistance when they identify plots in need of attention. In addition, by
training everyone in a specific set of practices, members can find support
within the group to monitor each other's plots. This is particularly help-
ful in a community where half of one's land may be located more than
an hour from one's home and a couple days of heavy rain or winds can
dramatically affect the condition of coffee plants. On the subject of the
advantages of being in the Organic Group, Doña Marcelina explained,

> The way I see it, I don't know if this is right, there is no envy amongst us.
> No, we help each other. For example, the older men will say to you, for
> example, in my case, the other day a man came who is in the Organic
> Group, and he told me, "Look," he said, "the growth in your plots is
> already looking good. They are this big, but they are meandering. Clean
> it up, because the vines are going to come around. You rip up the vines
> and the growth will be ruined." Oh, OK. So I told my father. "He said
> the vines have already started to climb in the new growth." "Oh, OK.
> Right," he said. And this week it will be cleaned up. They come to tell
> you what you have to do in your plots. They advise you.

This kind of weeding, or *la limpia,* is one of the most laborious tasks in coffee production. For each coffee plot, days at a time, several times a year, are dedicated entirely to clearing vines away from the tops of coffee plants and clearing the ground around the roots of small growth that would otherwise leach the soil's nutrients. However, much time can be saved with an early warning from a *promotor* such as the one Marcelina describes.

In conventional production on a large coffee finca, shade trees are nonexistent, precluding the problems of parasitic vines, and low growth is cleared though herbicide application. Bella Vista residents were accustomed to the use of herbicides from their time working in fincas at lower elevations. But in the steep slopes of mountainous coffee growing regions, where prized coffee such as that of Bella Vista grows in limited quantities, the consequences of herbicide application are grave and enduring. Herbicide application strips the soil of any ground cover. Then when heavy rains fall, as they do annually from May through September, the unprotected soil washes downhill, compromising the roots of the coffee plants and slowly diminishing the amount and quality of the land, a precious and hard-won resource. Though manual clearing of the land by machete is significantly more time consuming, most residents in Bella Vista view the work as a worthwhile investment in their coffee plots. An unknown number of members of the Conventional Group have attempted to make clandestine herbicide applications, but the majority of members in both groups have reprimanded and penalized those offenders. Through selective clearing, they are able to preserve a sufficient amount of ground cover to protect the root system and prevent erosion.

In addition to protecting roots and preventing erosion, manual clearing allows residents to plant small amounts of food crops alongside their coffee plants. When the residents of Bella Vista were living on conventional coffee fincas, they were not the owners of the land they worked, nor were they permitted to use the land for any purpose other than coffee production. But many of the small plants considered as weeds by finca owners, only to be eliminated with chemical herbicides, are actually edible or medicinal. In fact, when household funds are tight, families may forage for edible plants to supplement their meals. Using manual weeding techniques, coffee growers may plant squashes, greens, fruit trees, even corn to grow symbiotically with their coffee plants. As a result, while weed control through chemical application presents a quicker and easier solution, for a large number of residents of Bella Vista, the additional benefits of manual control—soil preservation and edible plants—make the organic method worth the additional effort.

Another crucial element of organic production, biological pest control,

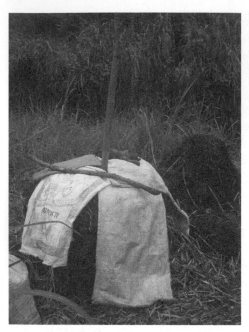

Figure 3.4.   To build bokashi, a method of composting, layers of chicken excrement, brush, trimmings, ash, and more brush and chicken excrement are covered in sacks to facilitate decomposition.

has proven so useful that Conventional Group members continue to use the techniques they learned from Toro Verde. *Broca*, or the coffee borer beetle, was among the most problematic insects reported by community members. Coffee borer beetles reproduce by boring into the coffee cherry and laying eggs. Once the larvae emerge from the eggs, they eat their way out of the coffee cherry, thereby destroying the fruit. According to the University of Hawaii at Manoa (n.d.), "Three types of damage have been reported: 1) premature fall of young berries, 2) increased vulnerability of infested ripe berries to fungus or bacterial infection, and 3) reduction in both yield and quality of coffee, reducing the income of coffee growers."

Toro Verde has imparted to Bella Vista residents several methods of *broca* control, including the popular *broca* trap. The trap consists of a 2-liter plastic bottle painted red, below which hangs a capful of methyl and ethyl alcohol. The color of the bottle and aroma of the alcohols attract the pests, drawing them into the liquid. When the insect becomes drunk on pure alcohol, it falls into a basin of liquid soap below, so that it is trapped and cannot escape. Though professionally manufactured *broca* traps are available for purchase, Toro Verde offers workshops on do-it-yourself construction of the traps, which have proven so effective that nearly everyone in the community makes their own and uses them in their plots. As a benefit of their partnership with Toro Verde, the Organic Group

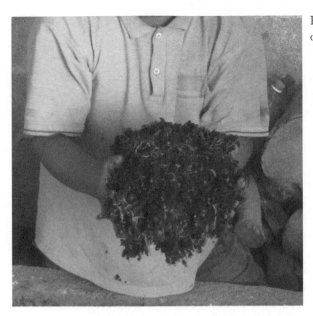

Figure 3.5. Handfuls of Red wrigglers.

members also receive donated supplies to construct *broca* traps for their coffee plots. Though Conventional Group members do not receive any support in purchasing materials, they continue to assemble these traps using their own supplies.

For the most contentious practice of organic production—the manufacture and application of organic fertilizer—Organic Group members also receive support from Toro Verde. Organic fertilizer can be produced in-house with common household items, but the process can be time consuming and requires a fair amount of dedicated space. As one resident explained, "The advantage is that to work in organic production you can find the inputs or fertilizers in your same plot of land. Everything in the mixture—the sticks, the ash from the home, everything. With that you can make your own fertilizer. But it is a big job. It takes a lot of work."

Even when one dedicates the time and space necessary to produce organic fertilizer, the amount needed for coffee production would be difficult for an individual to produce. For example, if residents were to follow best practices to cover their coffee plots with adequate fertilizer, the average cooperative member in Bella Vista would require 100 quintales of fertilizer for their land holding of 15 cuerdas. None of the residents in Bella Vista come close to applying this quantity of fertilizer. On average, members of the Organic Group apply 10 quintales of fertilizer to their plots, and even this quantity would be difficult to produce on one's own.

To bring them closer to best practices in coffee cultivation, Bella Vista residents received training and start-up funds from both Toro Verde and the national coffee association, Anacafé, to build a vermiculture facility. Donations of cement blocks and red wriggler worms were used to establish what has become an important source of fertilizer in the community. The project uses coffee pulp, a byproduct of processing coffee cherries, to feed the red wrigglers, who digest the pulp and excrete nutrient-rich soil as well as liquids that are used as a foliar fertilizer, sprayed directly onto coffee plant leaves.

The vermicompost project is highly esteemed by the community, as it is viewed as a self-sustaining, natural process, primarily reliant upon materials acquired from within the community. Residents pay a subsidized "symbolic cost" of US$2.56 (20 GTQ) for fertilizer purchased from the vermiculture project, though production is not yet sufficient to meet the rising demand within the community. In 2010, the vermiculture project was projected to produce sufficient fertilizer to supply 60 percent of the demand in the community, leaving some residents to continue purchasing supplemental fertilizer outside the community. Toro Verde often donates quintales of fertilizer to Organic Group members in order to support their new coffee plantings. Encouraged by the success of the vermiculture project in Bella Vista, both Anacafé and Toro Verde have pledged additional materials and funding to double the capacity of the facilities.

In the absence of chemical fertilizer, the organic cultivation system relies on plot renovation as a means of boosting production. In a coffee finca as old as Bella Vista, entire landholdings need to be renovated in order to have a significant impact on production volumes. To support the renovation effort in Bella Vista, Toro Verde also offers organic producers an annual donation of coffee plants to replace the old and tired trees in their plots. In 2010, members of the organic group in Bella Vista received 100 plants per household of their choice of coffee varietal. Fertilizer application is most crucial in the first three years of growth of the coffee plant, and beyond the initial investment in seedlings, the costs of coffee plot renovation in the organic system are considerable, including intensive labor to dig exceptionally large holes, sufficient organic fertilizer to fill these deeper and wider holes, as well as the transportation of fertilizer to remote coffee plots.

The organic cultivation system is rife with such examples of hidden costs of production. In another example, organic certification dictates that the time-sensitive task of coffee picking must be performed repeatedly, selecting only the reddest cherries and leaving the orange, yellow, and

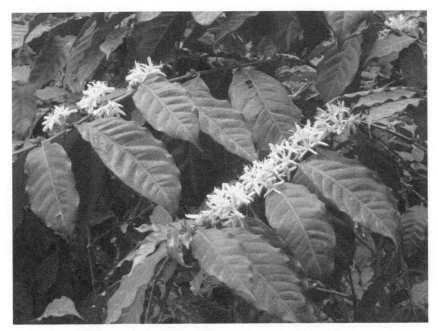

Figure 3.6. White flowering coffee trees.

green cherries to continue to ripen. Such careful picking ensures that the farmers maximize their harvest of cherries at the peak of ripeness, resulting in the highest possible quality which will, ideally, fetch a higher price with foreign buyers. It also, however, results in a greater investment of labor, as coffee growers make endless passes over the same plots, ideally every fifteen days, carefully inspecting each and every cherry.

Unfortunately, these hidden costs of production pose a significant financial burden to farmers who are already struggling between annual coffee harvests. Coffee production only reaps one harvest per year, granting farmers a brief window of time during which they receive an income for coffee. In Guatemala, coffee is not usually ripe enough to be picked and sold until October, and production tapers off sharply in December. In the months between December and the following October, families dependent on coffee profits cut corners and make sacrifices to pay their household expenses such as food, education, and medical costs. Rarely do farmers find themselves with disposable income to dedicate to upgrading their coffee plots. As mentioned above, this burden weighs especially heavily on organic farmers, who face even greater delays upon receipt of their annual payments.

In order to help organic growers invest in the future of their coffee production, Toro Verde offers prefinancing, wherein farmers can borrow money at low interest rates to cover the costs of planting during the

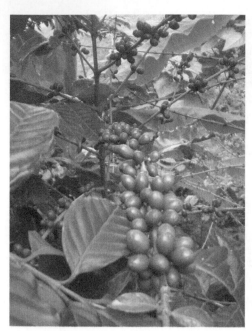

Figure 3.7.   A branch of cherries.

financially barren months of the year. Bella Vista's Organic Group members can request loans of several thousand quetzales to spend on cultivation-related expenses such as seedlings, fertilizer, and labor. In a survey of 2008–2009 coffee production practices (Dowdall 2012), residents in Bella Vista reported the following expenditures: fertilizer (Organic Group – US$25.64 [200 GTQ], Conventional Group – US$28.59 [223 GTQ]), hired labor US$192.31 [1500 GTQ] in both groups, seedlings (Organic Group—0 GTQ, Conventional Group US $44.87 [350 GTQ]).

Once the coffee profits are returned to the community, deductions are made and accounts are settled before farmers receive their final take-home pay. Conventional Group members also have access to loans through their cooperative, though many indebted members have evaded repayment by selling their coffee outside the cooperative altogether, thereby damaging the strength of their cooperative, both in terms of cohesion as well as financial resources.

Factors influencing cooperative membership

The support that the umbrella organization Toro Verde offers has allowed the residents of Bella Vista to overcome a number of obstacles that typically stand in the way of organic coffee cultivation. While many agriculturalists in Guatemala are unaware of the principles of organic production, Toro Verde provides training in new cultivation techniques. Moreover, it equips members of the community with knowledge to assist each other in best practices for coffee growing. Though coffee growers struggle to weather the financial burden of transitioning to organic production, Toro Verde donates supplies such as *broca* traps, seedlings, and materials to build an organic fertilizer facility, thereby easing the economic impact of the initial conversion costs. Though donated materials alone are not sufficient to cover all the coffee growers' needs, Toro Verde further assists growers by preparing them to produce their own fertilizer using materials available within the community, which lessens the cost of acquiring supplemental materials. While pest and weed control pose significant challenges to organic coffee production, organic farmers in Bella Vista have come to appreciate the longer-term benefits of their more time-intensive techniques, where the beneficial insects attract birds and other wildlife, and edible plants can coexist alongside coffee plants. Furthermore, Toro Verde established trade agreements with purchasers in the United States who are sympathetic to the precariousness of coffee production and willing to support farmers in the inevitable event of a natural disaster, thereby alleviating some of the economic risk of investing heavily in an agricultural activity. Finally, while sharp increases in labor and materials costs may impose considerable costs on farmers transitioning to organic cultivation, the opportunity for prefinancing through Toro Verde allows farmers to make significant investments in their coffee plots that will pay off in increased productivity in two to three years' time.

Additionally, the transition to organic coffee production can be linked to a number of indirect and unanticipated positive developments in the community of Bella Vista. Partnership with the umbrella cooperative Toro Verde has drawn the attention of a variety of NGOs based in the nearby city of Quetzaltenango. Now identified as a successful recipient of development support, Bella Vista has enjoyed increased traffic from development volunteers offering courses in a variety of skills such as tailoring, hairdressing, cake baking, and wood carving. Humanitarian tourists to the city who are interested in learning more about organic coffee production become acquainted with Bella Vista at the suggestion of Toro Verde and devote days or weeks of their travel to the community's new ecotourism project. While touring the coffee plots and production facilities, some tourists have become so inspired by the ambition of Organic Group members and ecological diversity of the coffee-growing jungle as to pledge additional support in the form of scholarships for children, basic medical training, English lessons, and funds to build a lodge for tourist groups. Riding high on their enthusiasm for the benefits of working cooperatively, a group of about twenty residents has organized to form a sustainable community development organization. In addition to their labor in the coffee plots, paid labor outside the community, and responsibilities to run a household and raise a family, these volunteers dedicate their spare time to clearing trails throughout the hillsides and building and maintaining the lodge for housing ecotourists.

But for all the apparent benefits of partnering with Toro Verde, the existence of a splinter Conventional Group indicates that some hurdles remain between the practices of coffee growers and the requirements of organic certification. In fact, upon seeing first the coffee seedlings, organic fertilizer, and *broca* traps delivered to their neighbors' houses, some members of the Conventional Group have grown resentful of Toro Verde, as they see these actions as a disregard for the economic hardship that they, too, are facing in their struggle to survive as coffee growers. The support of Toro Verde has allowed half of the residents in Bella Vista to feel successful and effective as organic coffee growers while the other half of the community still sees organic production as unattainable, ineffective, or unbearable.

Family size and structure

Among the Organic Group, there is a belief that organic producers are simply harder workers while conventional producers are less inclined to spend time in their coffee plots. Certainly the organic production method requires a significantly greater investment of labor, but for many households the availability of family labor to assist in the coffee plots is a tremendous help that makes this transition possible. Labor is needed throughout the year to weed, trim the shade trees, plant seedlings, and apply fertilizer. From October to February, farmers need as many hands on deck as possible to make the careful and repeated passes required to meet the strict quality standards of organic-certified coffee picking practices.

Large families, younger heads of household, and families with extensive local networks are better equipped to meet such labor demands. Able-bodied heads of household can independently care for as much of the weeding, planting, and fertilizing tasks as they are willing to complete themselves during the cultivating months of the year. During the coffee harvest, any children over ten or so years of age can help to pick coffee beans with their families. Conveniently, the coffee harvest season coincides with Christmas vacation in Guatemala, so even older children who otherwise reside in the city to attend high school are available to help during this labor-intensive time of year. Large extended families can collaborate to make relatively quick work of the coffee harvest and assist in big planting or weeding jobs.

The family surrounding Doña Marcelina enjoys all these advantages in production. Though she only has four children, compared to the average of six children per family in Bella Vista, they range in age from twelve to twenty-one, and all help in the coffee plots. Widowed at thirty-six, Doña Marcelina tends to her own landholdings as well as those of her brothers and sisters while they work as teachers and security guards outside the community. During the coffee harvest, all the capable members of the family organize to clear the coffee plots of one household at a time, comprising a crew of as many as twelve pairs of hands at a time.

In Don Efraín's case, however, he is solely responsible for all the labor in his coffee plots. His three daughters have all married and now manage their own coffee plots. His only son has been living and working in the United States for the past six years. His grandchildren are all under the age of eleven, rendering them too young to be of much assistance in the coffee plots. Barely managing to maintain productive coffee plants in the techniques that are second nature to him, Don Efraín does not feel that he alone can shoulder the additional labor burden of organic techniques.

Education and income-earning opportunities

Many members in the Organic Group sympathize with Don Efraín's struggle to keep up with time-consuming organic production techniques. Not all members of the Organic Group have such extensive families as Doña Marcelina, at the ready for help in the fields. For younger, smaller, or less able-bodied families, the most common manner of coping is to hire additional laborers to help with time-sensitive and labor-intensive tasks such as planting, weeding, and harvesting. To cover these expenses, Organic Group members hold an advantage in their more structured access to credit in the form of prefinancing, but many also have additional sources of income. In fact, 50 percent of Organic Group members that we surveyed were employed in some form of off-farm labor, often as security guards, teachers, and construction workers. Among Conventional Group members, however, only 17 percent of survey respondents held off-farm employment. Organic Group members, then, may be in a better position to subsidize the additional costs of organic farming with a steady cash flow of additional income.

Education levels may serve to explain in part the difference between off-farm employment opportunities between the two groups. Most positions in the nearby cities require basic mathematical skills and literacy of their employees. Within the community, 81 percent of Organic Group members had attended some school, compared with only 50 percent of Conventional Group members. Among those who had attended some school, Organic Group members reported completing an average of seven years of schooling, indicating some post-elementary education. Conventional Group members, on the other hand, reported completing only about four years of schooling, considered the bare minimum to develop basic literary and computational skills.

It is also important to note the considerable age difference between members of the two groups. Among survey respondents in Bella Vista, the median age for Organic Group members was forty-two compared with fifty-four years of age for Conventional Group members. Younger residents benefitted from educational opportunities within the community. Their parents, on the other hand, likely never had attended school or received a quality education on the coffee fincas where they were raised. As a result, the employment opportunities available to Conventional Group members are much more limited than those available to the younger, more educated Organic Group members. The availability of alternative income-earning opportunities, in turn, relates to a farmer's ability to subsidize the transition to organic production and cover basic household costs while waiting months to receive coffee profits through the organic repayment system.

Independence and liberty to work

All financial and time constraints aside, a more profound reasoning belies the Conventional Group's decision to cut ties with Toro Verde. After so many years working as day laborers on the coffee fincas of their past, the residents of Bella Vista place great value upon their liberty and independence as landowners. They no longer follow an owner's orders. They are free to work according to their own schedule. They can choose to invest more or less time in their coffee plots in response to other income-earning opportunities that may arise. They may be more or less attentive to their fields depending on their financial resources, availability of family labor, personal health, and any number of the infinite variables considered in the complex calculus of coffee growers' household expenses.

The organic system, however, and organic certification in particular, require coffee growers to follow a regimented work schedule and document their actions in a registry to be submitted for inspection by certifying parties. As the leader of the Organic Group explained,

It takes a lot of patience to work with so many documents, and the people are also really bothered that they have to maintain a registry of what they do each day. "And today I worked in the plots. And "today I cleaned." Or "today I pruned." Or "today I trimmed something. Then I added fertilizer to everything." You have to make a note of it. It is a lot of work and it is difficult but we want a good price, so we have to do it.

For many residents in Bella Vista, the requisite documentation presents not only another tedious task quite unlike the familiar physical demands of coffee cultivation, but, more than that, it represents a yoke on their freedom to work as they please. By following someone else's work schedule and maintaining a record for review by an outside party, many residents feel that to work under terms of organic certification is to forfeit the very independence they struggled so hard to achieve upon settling the community some thirty years ago.

In a panic over the internal struggles regarding how best to cultivate and sell their coffee, one member of the Conventional Group called upon the original priest who helped establish the community. The priest reacted by traveling back to the community to remind residents of the original purpose of their settlement. One resident related the story:

> … he said, "Guys, here no one is going to tell anyone else what to do. I brought you here to be free, to grow coffee, *pacaína* (date palm) whatever in your plots. It's yours and no one is going to tell you what to do there. If you want to apply [chemical] fertilizer, you can. You're free." So we in the Conventional Group are happy because we are free in our work in our coffee plots. To grow what we want. That's where we are. The other group, if they are happy doing what they're doing, great. They're free. That's where we are. Now you know why there are two groups.

Rather than view organic production as a long-term investment in the future of the community, many Conventional Group members view the requirements and restrictions of organic certification as just so many constraints designed primarily for the benefit of consumers in developed countries. They feel they are asked to take precautions and make tremendous sacrifices for the benefit of consumers up north and to the detriment of their families' needs.

Persistent short-term needs lead to persistent chemical use

A divide still remains between the two groups in Bella Vista. But the factors that separate those who feel that the organic system is worth the additional effort from those who remain unconvinced are many and varied. On the one hand, half of the residents in the community place a high priority on environmental preservation, are willing and able to take on the extra work of organic techniques, and appreciate the non-monetary benefits of working in the organic cooperative. The other half of the residents, however, feel greater pressure to address immediate household needs, find unbearable the sacrifices in production that seem to be an inevitable result of organic techniques, struggle to reallocate the time and labor needed to maintain organic certification, and bitterly resent the hoops they would have to jump through to access the benefits of being in the Organic Group. For half of the residents in Bella Vista, a complex combination of needs renders any risk taking in production infeasible and irresponsible to their immediate well-being.

For the Conventional Group members who have not yet applied chemical fertilizer, rejoining the Organic Group is a mere matter of re-applying for certification and submitting to the requirements of organic practices. For those who have applied chemical fertilizer, however, returning to organic production has become next to impossible. These farmers would have to invest in the time and labor of organic practices for a three-year transition period without receiving the full benefits of selling certified organic coffee. And the incline of this uphill battle only grows steeper with time as farmers continue to apply chemicals. The land demands more and more fertilizer to produce the same results, and the goal of transitioning back to organic becomes increasingly elusive.

Organic coffee production requires a significantly greater investment of time, labor, and financial resources compared to conventional production. Virtually all stages of production—acquiring organic seedlings, planting, fertilizing, weeding, picking—become more labor intensive using organic techniques. Organic producers are encouraged to increase their productivity by renovating their coffee plots, purchasing new seedlings and installing them with large volumes of fertilizer. And for coffee growers who have been growing conventional coffee for decades, new production methods require training and reeducation in totally unfamiliar methods of production. Meanwhile, the international market for coffee encourages producers to supply ever-greater quantities of coffee while minimizing the natural variation that is an inevitable result of production without chemicals.

In the midst of market pressures to continually intensify coffee production, some residents of Bella Vista have found a way to make chemical-free ecological coffee production a lucrative and sustainable enterprise. The umbrella cooperative Toro Verde offers materials, training, and credit to offset the hidden costs of transitioning to organic. Members receive donated seedlings, fertilizer, and *broca* traps to renovate their coffee plots. They participate in workshops to learn best practices in the organic system. Access to low-interest credit allows farmers to shoulder the costs of hired labor and material costs as they await higher-volume coffee harvests. Without this support, organic coffee production would never be an option available to the residents of Bella Vista.

The examples of Doña Marcelina, Don Efraín, and their families serve to illustrate the complicated picture of organic coffee production in the Highlands of Guatemala. The residents of Bella Vista overwhelmingly disapprove of the use of agrochemicals. They condemn the air and water contamination they see as a result of chemical use at lower elevations and boast of the purity and natural beauty of their mountainside community. They have some awareness of the health and environmental hazards associated with agrochemicals, and even those who practice conventional cultivation techniques strive to minimize their application of chemical fertilizer. But despite all the intention and desire to refrain from chemical use, some residents of Bella Vista do not yet feel they have found a feasible alternative.

Instead, they are entertaining the idea of incorporating additional agrochemicals—herbicides and pesticides—into their cultivation practices in order to gain a competitive edge and get ahead of their mounting household costs. Some farmers have gone so far as to apply these prohibited chemicals on the sly, stopping only when threatened with financial sanctions. The production advantages of agrochemicals only grow more tempting, as organic production does not provide an effective solution to the complex problems they face in keeping their household financially afloat. The further they persist down this path of chemical application, the more elusive the possibility of quitting becomes and the deeper the farmers are drawn into the treadmill of immediate needs.

Unfortunately, the long-term effects of putting out so many fires in the short term have taken their toll on the future of coffee growers' families, communities, and country. The demands of chemical use divert farmers' time and energy away from long-term investment in the health and education of their families as well as the environmental protection of their community. As a result, persistent chemical use can be seen to have a negative impact on the well-being of Guatemala as a whole, as it continually saps the country of its potential for a healthy economy and whole cadres of educated leaders.

In the next chapter we will see that the concerns plaguing Don Efraín and Doña Marcelina are not uncommon; they recur throughout

Guatemala and throughout agricultural industries. Whereas this chapter has focused on the overarching pressures of immediate needs, the next chapter considers the factors that restrict farmers' options for meeting these needs, exploring the labor-time and knowledge-dependence treadmills associated with agrochemical use as well as some successful efforts at interrupting their momentum.

Chapter 4

Change Comes to the Valley: Confronting Agrochemical Use with Local Organic Food Systems

On a rare clear afternoon, we could gaze across the valley of San Carlos in Guatemala's western highlands and a varied landscape resembling a patchwork quilt. The hamlets situated in this valley, the primary site of our research on export vegetable farming, are surrounded by mountainsides carved into precise, square agricultural plots meticulously cared for by the valley's inhabitants. From the spaces between the small, roughly constructed homes of cinderblock and corrugated metal, extending outward to the doorstep of the gargantuan quarry, to the edges of mountain slopes, we see the evidence of small agricultural production. From this distance, a snapshot of day-to-day rural life in the Maya highlands quickly emerges.

Looking down into the valley, it is tempting to assume the small groups of indigenous farmers working the mountainside fields are completely insulated from the workings of the outside world. Rural life appears quiet, slow, and completely unchanged by time. However, even a brief chat with any San Carlos resident encountered along the dirt roads that crisscross the valley reveals that this assumption could not be further from the truth. Not only are the communities of San Carlos plugged into global processes through their use of cellular phones and cable television, but also their very work in agriculture is conditioned by overarching structures of global markets. It is this interface between local reality and global structures that shapes nearly everything in San Carlos, from family and community relations to household livelihoods, agricultural production, and even public health.

In this chapter, we unpack this meeting of the global and local through the work and public health experiences of the indigenous Maya export vegetable farmers of San Carlos. By focusing on the stories and perspectives of two farmers, we show how the trajectory of agricultural development in the valley has given rise to distinct processes that fuel the threats to public health presented by agrochemical exposure. We do that

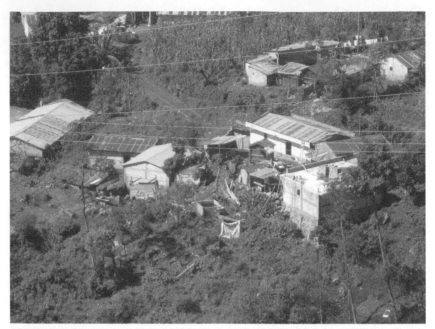

Figure 4.1.   A house on the mountainside in the Valley of San Carlos.

by extending the established metaphor of the agricultural treadmill to show how forces driving agrochemical exposure develop inertia of their own when combined with local circumstances. At the same time, while caught in a cycle that represents serious threats to their health, San Carlos residents remain active shapers of their own destiny. Far from passive, unwilling participants in a system that threatens their personal well-being along with that of their families and neighbors, many San Carlos farmers actively construct innovative solutions to the problem of toxic agricultural production. Highlighting their stories of setbacks and successes in confronting the health threats of agrochemicals, we show how a growing group of concerned farmers, local consumers, and supporting institutions have built social networks of collaboration and compromise to change cultural assumptions as well as the practice of non-traditional agriculture in the Highlands.

Livelihoods on the outskirts of a city

The northern valley of San Carlos is located in Guatemala's Department of Quetzaltenango, one of twenty-two political administrative units directly under the Guatemalan national government. The valley's moderate temperatures, ranging from 36–72°F, have made it an ideal site for agri-

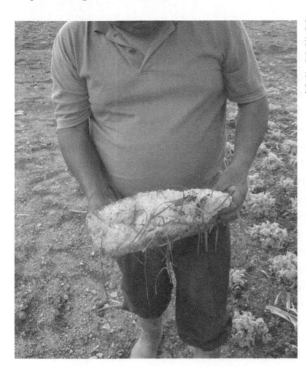

Figure 4.2.   A block of
ice chips that fell in a
hailstorm, destroying the
majority of this farmer's
leaf lettuce harvest.

cultural settlement since pre-colonial times. Its mild climate and strategic location made San Carlos an important center for the K'iche' Maya empire that held the region upon the arrival of the Spanish conquistador Pedro de Alvarado in the early sixteenth century. Even after Guatemalan independence from Spain, San Carlos has continued to serve as an agricultural center for traditional export crops such as coffee and sugarcane.

While moderate in terms of temperature, the valley contains wide variations in elevation, flora, fauna, and rainfall. Across the valley, elevations range from 7,545 to 9,514 feet above sea level, with average annual rainfall between 28 and 79 inches. The microclimatic zones existing within San Carlos are exposed to high variations in daily rainfall during the country's rainy season from May to October. Though the mountainous terrain offers some protection from hurricanes and other extreme weather, it is not uncommon for several days of downpour to be followed by several weeks of unbroken aridity. Such highly unpredictable weather patterns make the business of farming quite complicated for San Carlos residents, who confront unexpected pest outbreaks or topsoil runoff during periods of high rainfall and experience crop loss during periods of drought.

The ten small hamlets situated in the section of San Carlos where our study was conducted are home to just over ten thousand inhabitants. Though the valley has been populated by Guatemala's indigenous Maya population since pre-colonial times, in the first half of the 1990s the villages were established as politically incorporated cantons. Although each canton has its own democratically elected executive body charged with minor political administrative duties and general community leadership, most administrative decisions concerning infrastructure, public initiatives, services, and rural development in San Carlos lie with the municipal center in the nearby city of Quetzaltenango.

Unlike the nearby coffee-producing regions that are home to Bella Vista, the communities situated in the Valley of San Carlos are deeply tied to a neighboring urban center. Visible from nearly every hamlet in the valley, though often difficult to access via the narrow dirt mountain roads leading from the valley, the city of Quetzaltenango is a fundamental part of life for most San Carlos residents. A source of governance and employment for communities in the valley, Quetzaltenango is also home to numerous open agricultural markets where farmers sell their harvests to consumers and bulk purchasers. Not quite city residents themselves, inhabitants of San Carlos hamlets nevertheless maintain numerous connections to the city that impact their household livelihood strategies, agricultural production, and access to basic infrastructure.

Marginalization

Ethnically, little has changed in San Carlos since pre-colonial times. Of the total inhabitants of the valley, less than half of one percent is ethnically non-indigenous ladino. The remaining residents are indigenous Maya, many wearing traditional Maya clothing and speaking the K'iche' language in addition to Spanish. The majority of residents in San Carlos, like Guatemala's indigenous population as a whole, face high levels of poverty and economic marginalization as well as a lack of access to many basic services. Among our sampled population, average household size was 6.6 persons and average number of children per family was 4.65. Families of this size reported a median monthly income of about US$190 USD (1,500 GTQ). San Carlos families typically share two- to three-room structures, 93 percent of which have no system for wastewater removal.

Educational opportunities in San Carlos are sorely limited. In communities sampled for our study, adults reported having attended an average of 2.76 years of primary school. Studies of adult illiteracy in the cantons of San Carlos report averages ranging from lows of 25 percent

(ATQ 2001b) to highs near 80 percent (ATQ 2002). Though the majority of communities in the valley have at least one primary schoolhouse, children wishing to pursue education beyond the initial six years offered by such schools must travel between one and four miles by bus, or on foot, over mountainous terrain to urban Quetzaltenango. Because education is a significant added cost to San Carlos family expenditures, children often forgo schooling beyond the primary level to work on their family's agricultural plots or seek other forms of paid labor.

However, finding work can be a challenge. The lack of steady employment opportunities compels residents to combine a variety of small income earning strategies with farming, resulting in diverse household livelihood portfolios. Just over 64 percent of families living in San Carlos report holding at least one job in addition to agriculture. However, because agriculture is not sufficient to absorb the entire labor pool of San Carlos workers, many residents, particularly men, increasingly emigrate. The majority of households include at least one male member who works in construction, paid domestic work, or other manual trades in nearby Quetzaltenango. For these individuals, workdays begin with a thirty-minute to one-hour-long bus ride along roads that snake between mountain slopes and whose poor conditions make them impassible during the heavy rains of May to October. Other men opt to migrate internationally, leaving behind their spouses and children in search of work in the United States. Though reliable statistics on emigration from San Carlos are unavailable, a few observers and researchers working in the valley have noted the prevalence of an emigration scenario. According to one report (ATQ 2001a), migration is the third most common option for employment in one canton. Others (ATQ 2006) estimate that 50 percent or more of the male population of a neighboring community has migrated out of the village in search of work.

Scarcity of employment and education in San Carlos is matched by the lack of access of most community members to health care. All but two of the communities in San Carlos have no local access to medical treatment and services. The remaining two communities have makeshift health centers where outside medical personnel offer services at weekly or monthly intervals. In a scenario similar to that described by Filmer et al. (2000), most serious conditions requiring medical treatment compel residents to bypass these local clinics for more expensive treatments in Quetzaltenango. However, the costs of traveling to the city, coupled with the formidable fees charged for services in urban clinics, present San Carlos residents with a choice between two equally common solutions to illness: forgoing formal treatment to rely instead on folk remedies or undertaking treatment at potentially devastating financial costs.

Production of non-traditional agricultural export crops

Despite the diversity of employment and earning strategies in the valley, San Carlos households tend to engage in at least some farming activities, commercial or subsistence. *Milpa* cultivation (the planting of maize for household consumption) is the most common form of agriculture among farmers. Cultivation of a variety of non-traditional agricultural export crops—vegetables such as broccoli, snow peas, carrots, and radishes des-tined for supermarkets abroad—is also common. Farmers tend to divide commercial export vegetables and subsistence cultivation between plots of land. Though individual landholdings in San Carlos vary considerably, average farm sizes remain small at 1.7 acres.

Commercial farming is relatively new for most farmers in San Carlos. Much of what is known locally about this form of cultivation is a prod-uct of several decades of effort on the part of the Guatemalan government and various international actors to promote rural development and market integration of the Guatemalan countryside. Throughout the past several decades, the farmers of San Carlos, like a large proportion of Guatemalan farmers, have been encouraged by international and national campaigns to give up *milpa* cultivation and farming for home consumption and instead plant export vegetable crops for export to markets abroad. These efforts at rural economic development and agricultural modernization have fueled the rise of modern chemical based farming in San Carlos today.

The history of export vegetable promotion in Guatemala begins in the late 1960s in the realm of international development. Throughout the decades following the end of World War II policymakers and bilateral lend-ing institutions increasingly recognized that export diversification was nec-essary to revitalize impoverished rural Guatemala in the face of declining prices for traditional crops such as coffee and cotton on the world market (Fletcher 1970). International lending institutions such as the World Bank and IMF encouraged Guatemalan policymakers to promote increased cul-tivation of export vegetable crops such as snow peas and broccoli for sale in growing U.S. markets. According to planners, technological modernization of Guatemalan farms and the efficient production of export crops were the keys to economic growth and poverty reduction.

During the 1970s and 1980s, the United States Agency for Inter-national Development (USAID) was a champion of export agriculture in Guatemala, providing millions of dollars in loans to the Guatemalan gov-ernment to help foster export vegetable adoption. Drawing on existing models of the U.S. Cooperative Extension Service, export vegetable pro-motion programs involved the distribution of "packages" to farmers that included seeds for high-yielding varieties of commercial crops, synthetic nitrogen fertilizers, and chemical-based farm inputs. Accompanying the dissemination of these new inputs to farmers were seminars on how to apply the technologies and explanations of new farm management techniques for optimal crop yields. Developers also invested in export vegetable infrastructure, beginning with the introduction of ALCOSA, a vegetable exporting company that was a subsidiary of the U.S.-owned Hanover Brands Corporation (Brockett 1998: 52). ALCOSA received $17 million in USAID loans through the Latin American Development Corporation (LAAD) to purchase and export vegetables produced by Guatemalan farmers while implementing a massive agricultural technology-transfer to these small-scale producers (Brockett 1998).

Multinational involvement in and promotion of export agriculture continued in Guatemala into the 1990s and 2000s under favorable policies and promotion programs such as Highlands Agricultural Development, Trade and Investment, and Private Enterprise Development (Barrett 1995: 297). However, imports of Guatemalan vegetables dropped dramatically beginning in the early 1990s because large volumes of produce were found to have unacceptably high levels of toxic agrochemical residues and were detained at U.S. borders. Guatemalan producers lost approximately $20 million in earnings as their products were rejected at U.S. ports of entry between 1988 and 1994 (Thrupp et al. 1995).

The early 2000s saw gradual recovery of Guatemalan exports of key export vegetable crops such as snow peas. By 2003 Guatemala was again exporting over eighteen thousand metric tons of peas, eclipsing peak export rates from 1995 (Hamilton and Fischer 2005: 35). Though annual rates of growth steadily diminished between 2001 and 2005, export vegetables still accounted for 41 percent of primary sector production in Guatemala in 2006 (PNUD 2008: 125). More than twenty-three thousand Guatemalan households were involved in snow pea production alone in 2003, over 90 percent produced on stretches of land smaller than one hectare (Hamilton and Fischer 2005: 35). Small-scale farmers continue to supply intermediary exporters who then ship the aggregated product abroad from Guatemala City. However, prevailing quality standards of purchasing supermarkets now largely determine what exporters are willing or unwilling to purchase from small farmers.

Working to buy more time: Don Josue and POSC Organic Farmer Cooperative

Most residents of San Carlos belong to this small group of export-supplying vegetable farmers. Because high-yielding seeds for export vegetable crops were often distributed by promoters along with discounted chemical fertilizers and pesticides from the United States and Europe, adoption of export crops such as broccoli, carrots, and celery spread quickly among San Carlos farmers. Seeing an opportunity for quick economic gains, many farmers cleared all their lands and began planting export crops exclusively. The vast majority were far more cautious, portioning out one or two *cuerdas* of their total landholdings for commercial crops while keeping much of their land in *milpa* cultivation for subsistence. Still others did not adopt any commercial cultivation until several decades after the first introduction of these crops into the valley in the 1970s.

Among these late adopters is Don Josue from the San Carlos village of Comunidad de la Loma. We met and began working with Josue and a small association of export vegetable farmers called the Organic Producers of San Carlos (POSC) in 2007. Now the president of the group, Josue has been a major collaborator in our research into organic export vegetable farming. A fifty-year-old indigenous Maya man, Josue was born in San Carlos and has lived there his entire life. He currently resides with his wife and eight children in a small home just off one of the wider gravel roads leading into the valley.

In the past, Josue supported his family by combining a variety of paid jobs, including positions as a construction worker in Quetzaltenango and as a day laborer on numerous larger export vegetable farms in the area. Summing his occupational history, Josue remembers with a smile, "My work was always as a day laborer… a person who works doing whatever. The work didn't matter: plowing, weeding, I'd do whatever." Having only attended a few years of school before feeling the need to support his family, Josue found very little opportunity for employment in careers that required reading or mathematics. His situation is typical among San Carlos men. Reflecting on the diversity of employment options available to men in San Carlos he explains, "We are all construction workers. We work collecting garbage in Quetzaltenango. We're cleaners or bricklayers."

It was not until about ten years ago that Don Josue began carving out a couple of *cuerda*-sized pieces of his inherited lands to grow commercial vegetables to supplement his income as a paid laborer. Having learned a good deal about common farming methods and techniques from working on other farms, Josue first went to the local agrochemical store where owners eagerly sold him seeds, equipment, and chemicals for his newly cleared fields. Recalling his first few seasons growing commercial crops, Josue claims to have sprayed just about every available agrochemical onto his new crops. He remembers purchasing and dumping the contents of the bottles wrapped in red, blue, and yellow labels into his backpack sprayer. He rarely stopped to look at the long, complicated

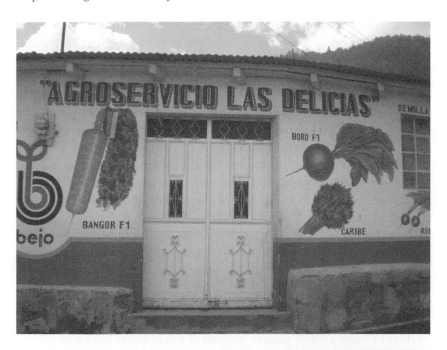

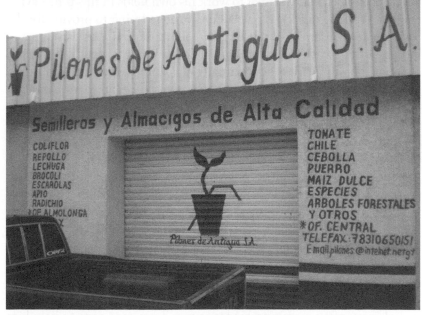

Figures 4.3 and 4.4. Agrochemical vendors and seed vendors of non-traditional agricultural exports (NTAE) in the Valley of San Carlos.

instructions or warnings on the bottles, instead preferring to spray these into the air everywhere around his new plants to ensure their protection. Just as he had learned working on other farms, Josue found that the best way to get new crops to grow quickly on his own lands was to spray more rather than less. Remembering those early times he recounts, "Sometimes a person uses chemicals and doesn't have the necessary knowledge… like what kinds of problems this can cause a person or the way these affect the health of each and every one of us."

Even before he farmed his own lands, however, Don Josue recalled several instances when coworkers would become suddenly ill in the fields, and have to sit down in the middle of the workday because of headaches or stomach sickness. Josue recalls, "I've seen it with my coworkers, because of the way we spray. And after, when we're finished spraying, we often get headaches…and what we used to do [as a remedy] would be to get some lemons and suck on those…because we believed that this would make it so we were unaffected by the poison." Though he and his coworkers often joked about the effects chemical inhalation had on their bodies, spraying chemicals quickly and carelessly had a very specific purpose: it allowed workers to cover a much greater portion of a field in far less time.

For Josue, it was essential to work his own fields in this time-saving manner. Working quickly is crucial for someone trying to provide for the basic needs of a family of ten by maintaining several jobs. Rising early in the morning each day to reach his first paid job at four o'clock, and continuing on to the next of potentially many other work sites afterward, Josue barely had any time to spare before the sun began to set. After returning home, with only a few short hours to work his fields before dark, spraying with chemicals became the only option available to him. To keep his farm functioning as a valuable source of income in addition to his other work and make a meaningful contribution to his family's survival, Josue needed to make his farming practices as efficient and failsafe as possible. To do so, he regularly applied huge doses of whichever chemicals were recommended to him by the local agrochemical vendors. Josue explains, "[I bought] whatever they sold in the agrochemical store and used it…I would rush home on days when I needed to work [on the household fields], buying chemicals or fertilizers. It was much easier to go and buy chemicals than to work organically."

Josue farmed his own fields in this chemically intense manner for several years, often recruiting his teenage and pre-teen sons to help him with big jobs. "They helped me a lot…. Yes, they planted seeds, worked the land, and yes, sprayed [chemicals]." Josue rarely considered the risks that spraying toxic chemicals without protective equipment, such as gloves or respirators, might have on himself or his family members. If he or one of his sons began to feel dizzy or experienced difficulty seeing while working, they would simply sit out for a moment or resort to a folk remedy such as lemon juice. While it was difficult spraying chemicals that he suspected had negative impacts on his family's health, Josue knew that this was his only choice, considering how difficult it was to manage his fields given the time constraints. Having to divide his time among several jobs, and with his sons in school and unable to dedicate much time to helping him in agriculture, Josue continued on this labor-time treadmill. He felt that undertaking the risks of chemical use for vegetable production was his only option.

It is possible that Josue would have never realized the severity of the threats that agrochemicals presented to his family had he not encountered a group of farmers from a neighboring village who introduced him to new ideas about cultivation and sales of export vegetables. This group, referred to locally as POSC, came to Comunidad de la Loma in the San Carlos Valley in 2006 with the help of a local NGO of agricultural scientists from Quetzaltenango. Josue remembers his first encounters with the group before joining,

> Before, I was really just a worker. I would look at how other people grew vegetables but I didn't know how to actually *sow* vegetables… what to apply to them or not, what kind of fertilizers, and how much to fumigate…. However, when they [POSC] came, they invited us to learn about how they grew vegetables…They soon began teaching us…about how when one uses these strong insecticides it contaminates the air we breathe…. So even if people are just walking by recently sprayed fields, it can affect their health as well as that of the environment.

In these early days of the POSC organic farmer cooperative, there was a core group of only about sixty farmers spread across three villages in the San Carlos valley. When Don Josue first encountered them, POSC was in the midst of recruiting new farmers in other villages by sending leaders and NGO agronomists to give local seminars about the dangers of agrochemical inhalation and exposure. Armed with a small projector and slideshow, POSC promoters came to Comunidad de la Loma in search of farmers willing to take a chance on a new way of farming and a new farmer-run microenterprise based on organic vegetable sales to local consumers.

By attending POSC seminars, Josue learned about a form of reduced-chemical farming referred to as agroecology, or more locally as "ecological agriculture," that relies on syncing agricultural production with local ecological conditions to protect natural resources and farmer health. More broadly, agroecology refers to an approach to agricultural systems that treats them as deeply embedded in the ecosystems and ecological processes of the surrounding environment. In practice, agroecology can involve myriad techniques and processes. However, such techniques generally focus on syncing ecological relations in agricultural fields with naturally occurring processes and organisms for improved production outcomes and minimal negative environmental and social impacts (See Gliessman 1998, Altieri 1995).

In contrast to the heavy-handed application of the latest chemical packages sold at the agrochemical store, this new approach to farming invited farmers to work together with agricultural scientists to develop alternatives to agrochemicals, using local resources and ecological processes to control pests or nourish fields. Josue learned about "polyculture," or the strategic planting of different types of crops in the same fields to ward off harmful insects and other pests. He explains,

> The real thing that helped me the most is that I was able to diversify my planting… One row of each product. And this helps to control insects. For example if there are insects and disease that like a certain crop but there is another that they *don't* like nearby, the combining of these plants [in a field] will cause the insects to look elsewhere for a place to live.

For Josue and many other POSC members, this cut down on chemical use, thereby reducing exposure. He explains, "Some farmers fumigate fields numerous times during the process from planting to harvest. However, when you sow mixes [of crops], one plant helps another. This is a huge difference between organic and chemical crops."

Another way in which Josue learned to reduce chemical inputs in agriculture was by making composted fertilizers using animal waste and brush from the nearby forests. POSC members and agronomists outlined the benefits of substituting composted fertilizer for nitrogen-based chemical fertilizers. The agronomists explained these advantages as they taught local farmers the process of constructing and maintaining compost heaps in their fields. Josue explains, "They taught us to make many kinds of fertilizers from [the waste of] just about any animals we have…chickens, cows, pigs." For POSC farmers, this helps to cut the overhead costs of farming. Josue told us, "This kind of fertilizer is much cheaper than chemicals….The weeds and leaves from the mountain are cheap, whereas chemical [fertilizers] would cost me about 250 quetzales [$31.98 USD] for 100 pounds."

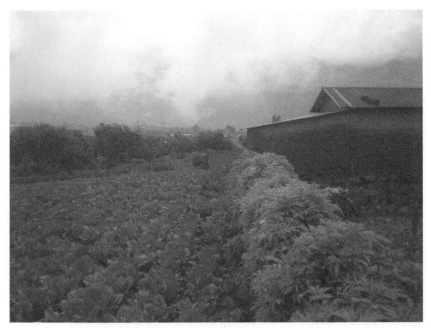

Figure 4.5. POSC farmer field planted in polyculture.

However, after joining the local chapter of POSC, Josue quickly realized that agroecology was a labor-intensive method of farming that required much more time than the few hours he was able to dedicate to cultivation. Like many POSC farmers, stepping out of this cycle of spending money to buy the time to earn more money was a formidable challenge. When asked about his transition to organic farming, one of the first things Don Josue had to say was, "[Organic farming takes] much more work because [with traditional farming] you only need to buy and spread chemicals. With organic farming, you have to prepare everything.... It's much easier to go and buy chemicals than to prepare organic [inputs]." This process includes hours spent weeding fields by hand and even setting natural traps for pests. To make matters worse, collecting leaf matter from the surrounding forests for composting often requires that POSC members carry awkward and heavy loads for long distances along narrow paths over extremely rugged terrain.

In many ways, the labor-time concerns of San Carlos farmers are similar to the issues faced by the Organic Group of coffee farmers in Bella Vista. Just as the organic coffee farmers found it difficult to dedicate the enormous amount of effort and time required for the making and applying of organic alternatives to chemical fertilizers, new POSC farmers face similar difficulties in their conversion to chemical-free agricultural

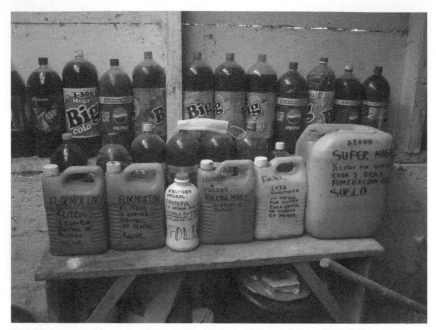

Figure 4.6.   A collection of organic fertilizers and pesticides made from garlic, chili, herbs, and animal urine.

production. While in Bella Vista, farmers faced a time sacrifice in hauling 100-pound sacks of compost to their remote fields, San Carlos farmers' diversified employment strategies left little time for hand-weeding fields or maintaining compost heaps. However, in both scenarios, farmers are easily caught in the undertow of chemical use and must swim against the tide in order to secure the long-term benefits of chemical-free farming over the short-term gains in productivity offered by chemicals.

In Don Josue's case, after a few trying years of hard work, he collaborated with POSC to develop a partial solution to the labor-time issue facing the majority of member farmers. A small composted fertilizer microenterprise was started under POSC control. Now, fertilizer production takes place via the efforts of dedicated POSC members, who then sell the compost to POSC in 100-pound sacks. The organization then resells the fertilizers to other members at production and transport cost. Josue explains, "Chemicals are a huge investment that cost farmers a lot. At the same time, with organic inputs…a person can easily make organic fertilizer, insecticides, and fungicides. That's easy. The real cost is the *time*. However, what helps is that one can now get these from POSC. They now bring together all of these organic things [for us]."

Don Josue has now worked with POSC for over six years and served as the organization's general president for the past several years. He is deeply involved in designing solutions to help member farmers escape the labor-time treadmill of chemical production and confront the public health threats of chemical use with low-chemical or organic cultivation techniques. Escaping the clutches of agrochemical dependence has proven to be a challenging task, but Josue is very optimistic about addressing the root causes of chemical exposure as they relate to the time and efficiency of agroecology and organic farming. He now works to arrange POSC activities internally so member farmers no longer have to choose between an efficient, manageable form of export vegetable cultivation and the health of their families and neighbors. Summing up his experiences with the labor-time demands of agroecology, Josue states,

> The difference [between organic and chemical-based cultivation] is that a person gains a consciousness about their own products and the awareness that their products are guaranteed to be free from chemical contamination and poisons. Sure, the work isn't easy. It's actually quite difficult because a person has to work hard to acquire the [organic] inputs. But we [POSC farmers] have achieved a lot in addressing this ... allowing people to get inputs without a problem. Organic still requires more work, but the differences between it and chemical-based cultivation are important.

Egoism and competition:
Doña Josefina and the women of POSC

One of the less positive, unintended effects of export vegetable introduction and market integration noted by the vast majority of farmers in San Carlos is the rise of what is referred to locally as "egoism." The farmers we consulted for this study frequently brought up the fact that their neighbors were all working to supply an already saturated market for export vegetable crops. With so many community members competing to grab the attention of purchasers, mutual mistrust and resentment of their neighbors' success has put a strain on social ties at the community level. Observers of indigenous Maya culture in Guatemala, such as Goldín (2009), have noted a negative reaction on the part of informants to visible accumulation of wealth or goods by other community members. Personal financial success for some members within Maya communities has historically been regarded by other residents as the result of possible pacts with evil spirits or other forms of immoral activity. Similarly, San Carlos residents that we consulted often accused wealthier neighbors of making their huge profits by collaborating with drug cartels, or trading in illicit goods.

In many ways, the competition brought on by export vegetable farming has fueled a general sense of mistrust and secrecy concerning farming techniques among export vegetable producers in the valley. San Carlos residents frequently lament the decline of collaborative farmer groups like associations and cooperatives, as well as the pervasive unwillingness of neighboring farmers to share their knowledge of successful techniques. Informants noted an increase in this inwardly focused "egoism" among farmers over the past decade, as more and more community members began cultivating export vegetables in an attempt to secure a piece of an already oversupplied market. One San Carlos resident described this situation to us by asserting, "If you ask someone [for advice about their farming techniques], they won't just say 'It's this that I applied' or 'I normally use this [chemical]'.... Each person now only looks after their own harvest of vegetables...because of egoism and because there is so much competition in vegetables."

With reported declines in farmer groups and sharing among neighbors of experience-based farming strategies, many export vegetable farmers in San Carlos seek advice about proper cultivation exclusively from chemical vendors and owners of agrochemical stores. The majority of our informants noted that this attitude can result in excessive use of chemicals, as salespersons have a vested financial interest in selling more chemicals. This circumstance sets in motion a knowledge-dependence treadmill, where the only way to address a problem in chemical-based agriculture is to seek out new chemicals and further advice from the agrochemical retailers. The only conceivable solution to one chemical's failings appears to be the purchase and application of newer and stronger chemicals. In this process, agricultural production becomes a result of the workings of chemicals that are poorly understood by the users. For most export vegetable farmers, knowledge of how to address problems like pest infestation is based only on a set of expectations for the performance of chemicals. Production of agricultural knowledge is divorced from farmer experience with local ecosystem functioning or shared personal insights.

Doña Josefina from the Comunidad de las Nubes in San Carlos found herself in this situation nearly five years ago. Now a POSC member and president of her community's organic farmer group, the forty-year-old single mother of three was pressured into taking up export vegetable cultivation on her own as a means of supporting her family. As is the case for many families in San Carlos, Josefina's household was broken up by her then-husband's attempt to find financial stability through emigration. However, unlike Josue, who found work in nearby Quetzaltenango, Josefina's husband emigrated illegally to the United States in search of work. Because migrant work is largely dominated by male members of villages in San Carlos, agriculture has increasingly become the domain of the female family members they leave behind.

Unlike some of her neighbors, who continue to count on the financial support of their husbands, Josefina was forced to assume full responsibility for her household's farming with very little help or prior knowledge of cultivation. Three months after finding out that her husband had arrived safely in the United States, his correspondence and financial support began to drop off. Months passed without any communication from her husband; Josefina concluded that she had been abandoned and gave up hope of ever seeing her husband again. Realizing that she needed to provide for her entire household independently, Josefina assumed the management of her family's export vegetable fields while taking on odd jobs as a domestic worker. Summarizing her situation and that of many of her female neighbors, she states, "We here [in San Carlos] are working women. This [is what] has helped us the most. In this community, almost every woman *works*. With our babies strapped to our backs, or very pregnant, we are ready to work and struggle."

Finding support as a new farmer was one of the greatest challenges for Doña Josefina in her initial years of export vegetable cultivation. She asked among her neighbors, seeking advice on proper planting times, how to ward off pests, and how to grow vegetables with the qualities sought by purchasers. However, she found her neighbors, with whom she was accustomed to speaking freely, suddenly tight-lipped and evasive concerning agricultural matters. She remembers her frustrations: "Here there are no people [from whom one may seek advice]. For example, if someone has a problem with agriculture, they can't just ask within the community…with other people…. Here everyone is separated. Everyone looks out for their own vegetables…how to sow them, how to harvest, and how to sell. There aren't really any groups among us."

For several years, Josefina simply purchased whatever small bottles the agrochemical vendor recommended. She rarely questioned the products that she was told to purchase. Even though she was unable to read the labels on most of the packages, the shop owner assured her that applying more was almost always better than applying less, and that applying chemicals before pest invasion or disease outbreak was better than trying to save an already infected field. Though applying so many chemicals was costly, Josefina never had a problem with worms, insects, or disease that could not be solved with the purchase of a new chemical.

However, after her children began periodically complaining of nausea after eating vegetables from her family's fields, Josefina slowly came to a realization:

> Sometimes, we would feel pains in our stomach after eating a carrot, for example. Why? Maybe there was nothing wrong with the preparation. Maybe it was that the vegetable itself was contaminated [with chemicals]. I began to realize the problem had nothing to do with preparation and that the vegetables were already contaminated by what they carried *within* them. Even when washed well, they still carry contamination.

Even after coming to this realization, Josefina had difficulty protecting her family. Seeking adequate treatment for chemical ingestion proved difficult. There are no medical facilities in Comunidad de las Nubes; the village is physically separated from the modern clinics in Quetzaltenango by several kilometers of mountainous terrain. In order to receive adequate treatment for chemical ingestion, Josefina would have to purchase tickets for an hour-long bus ride into the city. Once there, she would be faced with the added barrier of prohibitively high costs for a doctor's visit. For many years, minimizing her use of chemicals was an equally difficult task. Even though she wanted to protect herself and her family, Josefina was unwilling to risk losing an entire crop just because she failed to follow the chemical vendor's advice. She describes this dilemma, as well as the community and cyclic dimensions of the problem:

> When a person doesn't have experience sowing vegetables, advice comes from them [the agrochemical vendors].... How to address diseases, how to apply fertilizer, and the amount of chemical to apply. This [advice] often results in farmers using too much [chemical]. For this reason, a person needs to find a way to learn [about agriculture]....

> Our [bodily] defenses are already very low. What I see in my community is [people saying] "Why did so-and-so die? Because of some kind of disease..." But really, it is often because they have been [poisoned] by [chemical] fumes...What happens is that they prepare the chemical poisons and the aromas escape into their noses and lungs. For this reason, people often die of lung diseases. Why? Because of the poisons that they inhale while spraying....This hurts us as well but it has become the custom here...we *have* to spray.

With no personal knowledge of farming and no one willing to offer guidance, Doña Josefina found herself in a situation not unlike that faced by Don Josue or the coffee farmers of Bella Vista. As farmers with either no previous experience or possessing only prior knowledge of conventional, chemical-based farming techniques, all of these individuals were, in some ways, bound to the advice of chemical dealers and distributors. In the case of the Bella Vista coffee farmers and Don Josue, all previous experience with cultivation came from earlier employment on larger farms that relied heavily on the use of agrochemicals. Reversing the knowledge-dependence treadmill meant unlearning an entire system of cultivation. In Josefina's case, learning to cultivate export vegetables for the first time almost inevitably led her to the agrochemical vendor for instructions. Breaking dependence meant building new social groups with other local farmers in which knowledge of new forms of agriculture could be freely shared.

However, unlike the other farmers, Josefina faced yet another challenge to gaining control over the knowledge of agricultural production. Even though women in San Carlos increasingly serve as the principal agricultural laborers on their own lands, agricultural management and decision-making continues to be dominated by men. In San Carlos communities, characterized by the majority of our informants as *machista*, male-dominated societies, women learning about agricultural practices are rare. In fact, coping with machismo was a common theme among most women working in agriculture in San Carlos. While the notion of "machismo" can include widely varying social practices and behavioral norms across cultural contexts, the term is commonly used to describe a cultural bias favoring men and masculinity over traits and social roles ascribed to women that are considered feminine. Tracy Ehlers (2000: 7) describes the *macho* image to which many Guatemalan men conform as one of "unreliability, philandering, drinking, and wife abuse."

In this situation, Doña Josefina found it difficult to question the advice she received from the men at the agrochemical store. We asked Josefina about her early years farming alone and her experiences buying agrochemicals. She indicated that she had rarely asked questions or spoken up because she "was always so timid and full of fear." It was natural to just accept and apply whichever chemicals the men recommended, regardless of their potential effects on her and her family.

Doña Josefina continued in this way for several years before meeting POSC member farmers from another village. At the time, she was coping with the loss of her husband and attending free counseling services for single women provided by an NGO that was active in San Carlos: "Shortly after I separated from my husband, I went looking for…how should I say?…institutions supporting women. I began working with a group and they supported me by providing a psychologist…. Then they introduced me to this group [POSC]." Since she was the first farmer that they had met from Comunidad de las Nubes, the POSC members began working intensely with Josefina to organize a group of women farmers in the village. Integration into the first farmer group in her village was a life-changing experience for Josefina. It was then that "[POSC] began getting us [women farmers] together…and I had to represent my community to them. From that point I began losing my fears…. They called me and chose me [as the president of the local group] because they saw that I was becoming less timid."

The presence of a group of women organic farmers had numerous impacts on participants and the community as a whole. Group members now had a new forum in which they could discuss personal experiences with agriculture. In this way, the grip of knowledge-dependence was loosened because farmers were able to seek advice through community-based channels rather than solely through the advice of agrochemical vendors. Josefina describes this change as a process:

> [Previously] women had no opportunities [to learn about agriculture]. Now women are beginning to value themselves…. Their mentalities are changing. Working in an association causes us to wake up…. Now the agrochemical store is little more than a barrier, nothing more. Now we have the idea [of cultivation] ourselves. We have our own ideas of how to sow crops and how to control pests…. This is all part of the process.

At the community level, farmers now have a working social institution that, according to Doña Josefina, "forces you to communicate with others and to rid yourself of the egoistic idea that 'I have my crops and only I will sell them.'" For her, the presence of a group "has allowed us to learn together. If we weren't [working together] in groups, it would be more chemicals and only chemicals." As the local president of the POSC organic farmers of Comunidad de las Nubes, Josefina is now very active in organizing weekly meetings and seminars on organic farming for local members. She occasionally travels with the group to new communities to talk about organic export vegetable farming. She has also taken an active interest in her seventeen-year-old niece's education by integrating her into the group and helping her to rid herself of her timidity and fear of speaking through regular participation.

Getting local farmers to work together and share their experiences with agriculture has not been simple, particularly for women. Machismo and mistrust continue to present challenges to participation and learning about new forms of agriculture. Josefina laments the numerous women

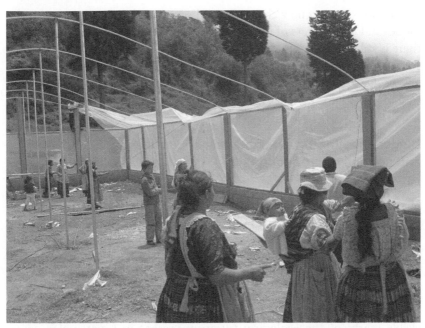

Figure 4.7. Their heads covered to block the midday sun, women of POSC gather to construct a greenhouse where they will grow seedlings for distribution among group members.

who would like to participate, but are unable to because their husbands disapprove, or are suspicious of their wives leaving the home: "Because there is still a lot of machismo, many husbands won't let their wives come [to POSC meetings]…and many women are left with little time to come to meetings [due to their work in the home]. They say, 'I don't have time to come.'"

Josefina admits that her situation is slightly different from these women: "If I were still with my husband, I wouldn't have learned all that I have learned [with POSC]. Because with a husband, a woman has to be in the home. She can't leave. Women often tell me, 'Our husbands won't give us permission to join groups.' And we never see them come."

In spite of these difficulties, Doña Josefina and many of her fellow POSC members in Comunidad de las Nubes have seen changes within their lifetimes that give them hope for the future. With many men in the community seeking paid work outside of agriculture, women have taken over a greater part of decision making concerning farming and a more public role in community affairs. The POSC members of Josefina's community see this change as an opportunity to bring in more members from the surrounding area and to spread the message about low-chemical agriculture, opening new channels for discussion about agricultural techniques and the dangers of certain agrochemicals. Though they admit that there is still much machismo and egoism within their communities, they see the growth of their group as a meaningful step toward addressing the knowledge-dependence treadmill that fuels community members' exposure to many harmful agrochemicals.

Bigger is better: urban consumers and notions of product quality

Chemical-free farmers such as Josue and Josefina face yet another complicated set of challenges when they bring their produce not sold through POSC to the open markets in Quetzaltenango. Most farmers competing in these markets are compelled to apply large amounts of chemical fertilizers and pest repellents in order to offer produce that attracts customers. Farmers who grow and sell organic, chemical-free export vegetables are in a difficult position because their products lack many of the synthetic fertilizers and pesticides that make them large, uniform, and free from visible marks of the ecological variation present in Guatemala's countryside. These differences make it difficult for POSC farmers to market their produce alongside its chemically treated counterparts. Expressing his frustration with trying to sell organic produce in local markets, Don Josue explains, "A product with chemicals looks like it is of much higher quality than an organic one. It looks juicier. The organic, on the other hand, looks like it is of lower quality...Even though the organic may have a much better flavor, the majority doesn't care about flavor. They instead only look at size." Josefina observes,

> It seems to me that the vegetables treated with chemicals are bigger. For example, the carrots and the onions.... Now, what was once seen as a normal size [for a product] is seen by consumers as small.... Our [organic] vegetables aren't contaminated. But, for this same reason, there are often people in the market where we sell in the city that say, 'Oh no. These beans are very small. We want the really big ones and these are small.' There are big ones but they're like that only because of the large amounts of chemicals used.

As we explained in Chapter Two, major supermarket chains that carry imported fresh produce have specific sets of standards for product appearance and freshness that favors the use of toxic agrochemicals among farming populations. In typical conventional export vegetable chains, standards for product quality are mainly enforced by local intermediary bulk purchasers, who buy vegetables from farmers that they resell to exporters in Guatemala City. Intermediaries from neighboring townships who arrange the purchase of export vegetable products are frequently the object of negative feelings among farmers. Referred to locally as 'coyotes,' export vegetable intermediaries are resented by farmers for their power to contract produce from individuals, only to reject it later because it does not meet export standards for quality. In conventional export chains this drives chemical use among farmers because they compete with one another using pesticides and fertilizers to provide the coyotes with the largest, most blemish-free, and most uniform produce.

Supermarket standards for produce quality are no longer restricted to international markets. According to many of the San Carlos farmers, the enforcement of supermarket standards for cosmetic quality of produce has begun to affect their ability to sell in local open markets as well. As chemicals become increasingly integrated into local production and markets, many consumers and producers have internalized these assumptions about product quality. Blemish-free, large, uniform, and perfectly symmetrical produce are the emerging local market and farmer standards for well-farmed produce. This gives rise to a quality-preference treadmill that develops momentum as irregular sizes and blemishes from local pests or differences in environmental conditions are presumed to be markers of low quality produce.

Farmers who base their household budget on earnings from sales of chemically treated produce cannot easily shoulder the risk of losing the income contribution of export vegetables that is brought on by changing methods of production and going chemical free. The engine of quality preference pressures farmers to continue spraying and influences consumers to buy only the biggest, brightest produce they can for their money.

Overcoming the prevailing notions of produce quality held by local consumers has been perhaps the most difficult task for members of POSC as they attempt to establish a microenterprise based on local consumption of chemical-free vegetables. In response, the organization has worked with a locally based NGO in the areas of product development, service, and consumer education in Quetzaltenango. The result has been the formation of a local food system based on direct marketing and weekly doorstep delivery of the group's flagship product, the Bag of Eco-Vegetables. Delivered by POSC farmers to over 130 consumer households in urban Quetzaltenango, the POSC Bag of Eco-Vegetables is the result of pooling members' produce that features ten or more seasonal vegetables. Bags are assembled in a POSC processing facility in San Carlos by paid members who trim and package the organic vegetables on a weekly basis.

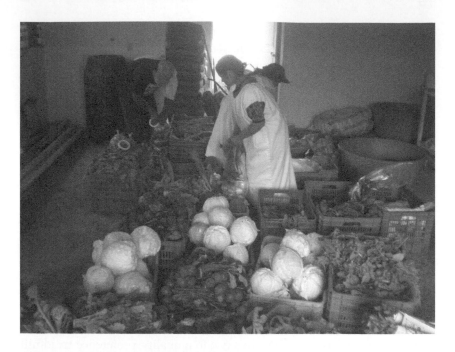

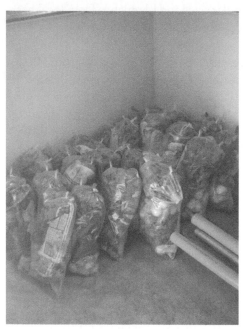

Figures 4.8 and 4.9.   Women dressed in sanitary gear pack vegetables from members' plots to construct the Bag of Eco-Vegetables.

Delivery of the Bag of Eco-Vegetables and the administration of the microenterprise have required more than just the development of novel products and services for consumers. For both POSC farmers and consumers, education is both central to success and a key limiting factor to the growth of the local organic food system. For many POSC farmers, human capital development has taken the form of member trainings in the Best Practices for Food Handling and Farm Management. Training for these certifications, maintained under the Integral Program of Agriculture and Environmental Protection (PIPAA) of Guatemala's Ministry of Agriculture, Food, and Livestock (MAGA), has familiarized POSC farmers with a basic set of procedures for food processing that ensure product sanitation.

While sanitation in food handling and processing have been relatively easy for POSC to ensure, efficiency in business administration has been elusive. Members like Don Josue see this as one of the greatest challenges to moving forward with the POSC enterprise:

> Right now we're really seeking out a better way. It's great that we're [POSC's leadership] meeting regularly to talk about our problems or needs and how to solve these.... We are capable [of directing the business] but it has been a little difficult. Maybe it is because of the lack of academic preparation among members…perhaps it's that we're not very well prepared. It's very difficult for us to make sense of certain kinds of information. Almost nobody knows how to use computers.... But at least the NGOs are giving us workshops in this area. For this reason, POSC remains highly dependent on support from outside NGOs, who continue to provide financial administration, accounting services, and coordination for the microenterprise.

Education on the consumer side has also been a central focus of POSC activities. One of the major objectives of the group is to spread the word among consumers about the dangers of ingesting foods that have been excessively treated with toxic agrochemicals. The battle has been uphill due to several interrelated factors, including low levels of awareness of the effects of agrochemical consumption and the economic hardship faced by even the relatively well-to-do, urban, middle-class that makes up the primary consumer base of POSC products. Unlike the coffee farmers of Bella Vista, who can receive higher prices from a growing consumer base for organic coffees abroad, POSC vegetable farmers have no way of accessing foreign markets for organic produce. Instead they are forced to inform local markets about the benefits of organic produce, one consumer at a time. Expressing his frustration with educating consumers Josue states,

In Guatemala, even though we would like to, we don't have a culture of quality for the products we sell. This is the question. You [the North American interviewer] know that a [chemical-free] product is less harmful to your health and so you buy it even if it is more expensive. You know that it will not harm you. Here people will buy a product even if they know it will hurt them simply because it is cheaper.

Growth of the microenterprise's consumer base has been a slow but steady process of educating each and every new consumer. POSC members like Josue and Josefina know that creating a larger market for their products among urban consumers is crucial for keeping their business alive. At an even deeper level, their ability to foster education and human capital development on both consumer and producer sides of the local organic food system is the key factor to overcoming the quality-preference treadmill and ensuring the future success of the fledgling microenterprise.

Many POSC members whom we consulted maintain considerable hope for the future of the enterprise, pointing out that newer, younger members have had better educational opportunities and preparation for carrying out the financial and administrative aspects of the business. But it remains to be seen what impact these newer members can have on consumer notions of product quality. They face a considerable challenge in redefining existing notions of product value among consumers focused on acquiring only the largest and most visually appealing food for what little money they have to spend on their households' meals. As Don Josue explains,

> No matter what, people don't think of the benefits of [chemical-free] produce. They only look at the price because they don't have the money to buy an ecological product [from POSC]. Looking at a chemically treated carrot and an organic one, they will buy the chemical one…because they see its large size. What they don't think of is that, the bigger the product, the greater quantity of chemicals that it may contain. The people have no interest in buying something that they can't afford.

Producer and consumer knowledge gaps fueling persistent chemical use

Member farmers of POSC such as Don Josue and Doña Josefina represent a small but growing number of residents in the Valley of San Carlos who have developed novel ways to address the treadmills that perpetuate chemical use among export farmers in this part of Guatemala. Their stories are an encouraging example of the ability of small farmers to secure the financial well-being of their families without endangering their own health or that of those around them. The POSC farmers that we consulted maintain a high degree of hope for the future of the organic farming enterprise under the control of their children and a group of younger, more capable farmers. Equipped with better educational opportunities and human capital to invest in the financial and organizational management of the business, there is much promise for the future of the POSC microenterprise under a new generation of individuals who depend, at least partly, on export vegetable farming for their household incomes. Also, awareness of the dangers of ingesting harmful chemical residues in export vegetable crops seems to be growing among Guatemalan consumers, as general access to information in Guatemala is spreading with internet-based technologies and satellite communications. This trend is likely to raise consumer demand and fuel future sales of chemical-free products like the Bag of Eco-Vegetables.

At the same time, the socioeconomic forces that drive chemical use continue to operate upon younger farmers with an even greater intensity. As Guatemalan rural household livelihood and employment strategies become increasingly diverse, commercial farming is likely to become one of many income-earning strategies maintained by rural dwellers. In such scenarios, future farmers are less likely to have the time to spend on labor-intense farming methods like agroecology or chemical-free organic cultivation. As was the case with Josue, frequent and hasty applications of numerous agrochemicals may seem like the only way to keep up this valued source of income, given the time constraints imposed by engagement in a multitude of simultaneous income-earning activities. As both men and women take on paid work in urban areas within and outside of Guatemala with greater frequency, farming will become more and more the domain of the inexperienced. Like Josefina, many farmers in this situation may come to depend on chemical salespersons for advice on how much and how many chemicals to apply to their crops.

Though the future is uncertain, POSC farmers like Don Josue and Doña Josefina demonstrate an inspiring dedication to addressing the public health threats posed by agrochemicals. Though they swim against the general current of chemical-based farming in San Carlos, they see themselves as victors in the long term. Don Josue concludes,

> It's for the youth, not for ourselves that we started this organization. We're looking out for the health of our children, right? It's for a future in which our children realize the goals that we set for ourselves

today.... May it never end. May it continue moving forward forever.... If not with me, with others. May it become more developed, even if I myself don't benefit from the result. It is just like planting a tree. I plant it, but sometimes I don't see the fruits myself. It is *others* who will reap this fruit.

Chapter 5

Conclusion: Program Recommendations and the Application of Ethnographic Research in Public Health Initiatives

The rapid growth in the complexity of commercial farming systems over the past several decades has spurred strategies for managing nearly every aspect of agricultural value chains—from farming practices to assuring the safety of agricultural commodities that reach consumers. In this book, we explored the reasons farmers are increasingly driven to use toxic agrochemicals that continue to pose serious threats to the public health of farming communities, even in spite of a host of regulatory agencies. The past twenty years have seen massive consolidation of the global trade in agricultural goods under a few large-scale buying firms located in the global north, giving rise to a form of competition that prizes stable and steady supplies of uniform products that must be delivered irrespective of unpredictable environmental and social forces. These buying firms strive to reconcile the variability inherent in agricultural production with the needs of global competition by enforcing quality standards that emphasize consistency, generification, and standardization of the products in their value chains. As a result, the drive to modernize agriculture has generated many innovations that have revolutionized farming by allowing for more predictable and efficient production.

The importance of uniformity and overall production volume has placed enormous pressure on suppliers—and ultimately on farmers—to use whatever means possible to make their products comply with purchaser demands. Modern agrochemicals have become a standard tool for achieving uniformity and volume: they have the allure of quick and bountiful production, insurance against unpredictable environmental conditions, resistance to pest attacks, labor-saving advantages that conform to household needs, and strong eye-appeal to suit customer preferences. Across the globe, agrochemicals have allowed many farmers to secure a place in their respective value chains.

At the same time, the ability to standardize production has come at a high price for many farmers. Though quality standards do not directly mandate agrochemical use, and sometimes explicitly oppose the application of toxic agrochemicals, in global value chains their use has the potential to endanger the health of a multitude of rural producers around the globe. Many farming communities situated in the developing world must contend with a crippling combination of weak regulatory regimes, marginalized populations, high poverty, an absence of basic medical infrastructure, marginal workers, and low levels of education. Together, these factors create high-risk environments for toxic chemical exposure and can themselves be threats to public health.

In spite of attempts by international organizations such as the WHO, UNEP, and FAO to regulate agrochemicals, farmers in the developing world continue to be exposed to banned chemical ingredients that are either still legally circulated within their nations' borders or part of obsolete stocks that are still sold in spite of global prohibitions. One reason is the lack of converging epidemiological evidence concerning the threats to human health posed by many legal and unregulated pesticide ingredients. This creates a state of uncertainty, allowing millions of pounds of pesticides to be circulated annually, despite their ties to significant health hazards. Another reason for continued exposure is the lack of understanding among farmers of the hazards of agrochemicals and the absence of adequate safety equipment; as a result of these factors, many farmers are exposed to unsafe levels of unbanned chemicals as well. Indeed, many farmers in our study reported having experienced symptoms of chemical poisoning from unrestricted compounds or those determined to present only minor threats to human health *when applied as recommended.*

Given this situation, programs designed to address the public health threats deriving from agrochemical exposure in the developing world tend to focus on agrochemical awareness among farmers, promoting lessons in proper chemical application, providing safety equipment, and disseminating alternative farming practices. However, as in the case of the Safe Use Campaign and other similar programs in Guatemala, a narrow focus on education and safety equipment is not enough to protect farmers. These programs offer much-needed instruction concerning the application of harmful pesticides, but the ample evidence of overuse and illness related to agrochemicals around the globe demonstrates that awareness alone is not sufficient to affect change in farming practices.

Awareness programs fail because they assume that lack of education and safety equipment are the primary drivers of toxic chemical exposure and because they treat farming as an isolated activity, divorced from the economic realities and sociocultural contexts of farmers and farming communities. Our ethnographic research demonstrates that on their own these programs cannot adequately confront the root causes of toxic agrochemical use. Instead, public health programs aiming to reduce small-farmer exposure to harmful agrochemicals must address the underlying drivers of chemical use that are sustained by broader economic and cultural processes, such as debt structures, global markets, education, household structure, egoism, marginalization, employment opportunities, and other factors outlined in this book and reflected through the prisms of the lives of Don Efraín, Doña Marcelina, Don Josue, and Doña Josefina.

Addressing the drivers of the pesticide treadmills

To understand the persistence of the threats agrochemicals present to the health of farmers and their communities in Guatemala, we have employed the concept of the treadmill—a familiar metaphor in agricultural research since Cochrane's (1958) seminal work on market prices and adoption of new farming technologies. Going beyond this early formulation, we extended the concept of the treadmill to sociocultural dynamics set in motion when a farmer integrates agrochemicals into his or her cultivation practices. By following the stories of farmers of two of the country's most important export crops—coffee and fresh vegetables—we highlighted several interrelated processes that lead many farmers to overuse and misuse toxic chemicals in their fields. Critically, we showed that they do so *in spite of their awareness* of the health threats posed by many pesticides and contrary to their desire to care for the long-term well-being of themselves and their communities.

Confronting the treadmill of immediate needs

Many coffee farmers are motivated, at least in part, to avoid chemical use because they aspire to enter the potentially lucrative organic markets. However, meeting production goals without chemical fertilizers is a long-term, laborious endeavor that conflicts with the short-term needs of many farming households. We saw that Don Efraín's immediate household medical expenses could not wait on the delayed payment system for organic coffees. We also saw that taking advantage of the short-term production gains offered by chemical fertilizer applications and the immediate payment schedule of conventional coffee markets initiated a treadmill of immediate needs and economic dependence. Don Efraín had little choice but to continue applying an increasing quantity of chemicals to his coffee plots with each harvest in order to maintain sufficient yields just to cover his growing household expenses.

Economically dependent on the short-term gains of chemical use and conventional market payment systems, farmers like Don Efraín find it nearly impossible to reinvest in the benefit of organic cultivation over the long term. Part of his difficulty is the nature of organic certification requirements. Should a farmer decide to apply chemical fertilizers in hopes of producing a bumper yield in a year of extreme need, she must demonstrate at least three subsequent years of chemical-free cultivation before being able to again acquire organic certification. During these three years, she bears all the risks of organic production with none of the benefits of the organic market. Meanwhile, the temptation to raise the ante by applying more chemicals to one's coffee that is destined for conventional markets is ever present, guaranteeing profits in the short-term while raising the costs of production in the long-term. Though Don Efraín did not resort to the application of pesticides or other agrochemicals, several Bella Vista farmers in the Conventional Group did expand their chemical application practices to protect against immediate losses to their principal source of income. With organic certification seemingly out of reach, the pressure was too great for these farmers to slip into dependence on toxic agrochemicals under the production-centered logic of conventional coffee markets.

To address the specific needs of farmers like Don Efraín, who are already aware of organic cultivation techniques and the threats posed by agrochemicals, public health programs must move beyond education and training in the simple mechanics of reduced-chemical agriculture to confront the underlying drivers of the immediate needs treadmill. Our ethnographic work and the experiences of small export farmers recounted in this book illustrated very clearly the centrality of economic risk in small farmer decision making, a concept also established in the field of agricultural economics (see Ellis 1993, De Janvry 1972). Don Efraín and other small farmers at the economic margins tend to follow a "safety first" principle with respect to economic security (Scott 1976: 15), seeking to shield themselves against economic disaster in the face of unforeseen medical or other household expenses. In this case, agrochemical use offers to farmers a kind of insurance against crop loss resulting from changes in weather patterns or pest outbreaks, while providing the added security of higher crop yields and income from sales over the short term. Even if market prices for their crops suddenly drop, farmers can protect themselves—to a degree—by offering more voluminous harvests made possible by heavy applications of chemical fertilizers and pesticides.

Programs attempting to disseminate new, reduced-chemical agricultural techniques will not be successful enough if they promote only the beneficial health outcomes of their programs. They must design interventions that incorporate economic assistance so farmers can bear the financial risk during the initial transition period, before adequate market infrastructures are established for such products. For farmers like Don Efraín, programs must include provisions to manage risk directly on two fronts: to manage unforeseen costs related to health care emergencies, educational expenses, food security, and other basic household needs; and to secure the farming enterprise against weather and other environmental contingencies.

Some researchers suggest that greater access to credit will help farmers to protect their households' economic viability during the adoption of new agricultural techniques (see Eswaran and Kotwal 1989). Ethnographic research, which offers a deeper understanding of farmer livelihoods, is central to assessing whether forms of risk management such as credit or microlending schemes are appropriate. Although initiatives like crop insurance or microloans can work in some instances, our research shows that it is not an adequate solution for all farming households. Ethnography reveals the increasing complexity of livelihood portfolios, including farm household budgeting, risk management, and the place of farming as an income-earning strategy. This research is crucial for choosing the proper tools to address the risks and uncertainties producers face in contexts as diverse as those we have explored.

Confronting the labor-time treadmill

In addition to securing immediate needs, the steady use of agrochemicals serves another purpose for small farmers: it saves time and minimizes labor. Many people in San Carlos and Bella Vista see chemical-free farming as a labor-intensive impossibility. Farmers in San Carlos who engaged in numerous income-earning endeavors struggled as they tried to break free of the labor-time treadmill—even though they understood that many of the chemicals they used presented risks to their own health and that of their families. In Bella Vista, chemical-based farming saved Don Efraín hours of work because he did not have to hand-weed his fields, compost organic fertilizers, or design natural pest repellents. Many others in his community found it disadvantageous to apply hundreds of pounds of organic fertilizer to their distant coffee plots in order to enter the organic market, which did not always pay higher prices than the conventional market. The labor-time treadmill ultimately fractured the coffee growers' cooperative, an institution as old as the community itself.

How can public health projects apply an understanding of these complex economic realities to actual interventions? How exactly can programs designed to build alternatives to chemically intense agriculture be tailored to the increasingly diverse household livelihoods of farmers? A crucial challenge is to design effective strategies to lower the time and labor expenditures required of farmers pursuing reduced-chemical or organic agricultural practices.

Fertilizer-producing microenterprises, labor-sharing farmer associations, or even the production and distribution of organic pest repellents can complement the time and labor demands of agricultural livelihoods, though the ways in which they support livelihood strategies may differ. Some farmers have found that marketing schemes for organic products create sufficient profits to make the labor investment in specialty agriculture worthwhile. Consequently, these individuals scaled back or eliminated other kinds of work, freeing more time for agricultural activities. In other cases, however, a farmer's portfolio of income-earning strategies may be relatively inflexible, and in these cases chemical-free agriculture will be feasible only with programs that reduce the labor burden of these methods. In their design phase, public health initiatives can conduct or consult ethnographic fieldwork to identify the variety of household development goals in their target communities. Determining whether farmers engage fully in agricultural pursuits or need to minimize agricultural labor and reinvest time in other activities will guide the appropriate strategies to support these objectives.

Ethnographic methods are beyond the scope of this book, but we will emphasize one overarching point about the community research that should inform public health programs. Because of the context-specific nature of agrarian household economics, designing programs that effectively manage the increased workload of reduced-chemical farming requires farmer participation at every step of the project's development. As advocates of "farmer first," and participatory development projects like Robert Chambers (2007: 3) have stressed, establishing two-way knowledge flows between farmers and developers in the development process is the only way that programs can begin to account for the, "local, complex, diverse, dynamic, uncontrollable, and unpredictable realities experienced by many poor people." Public health also has a strong and growing body of community-based participatory research methods that should undergird this work (Wallerstein and Duran 2006, Israel et al. 1998, Eng et al. 1990.

In both of the communities we came to know in this book, chemical-free cultivation persevered, in large part due to the collaborative efforts of farmer-led organizations and agricultural program designers. In each case, substantial labor required to produce organic fertilizers was addressed with labor-saving projects such as vermiculture or composting enterprises that drew on resources available to farmers in their respective communities. Though neither project has been a panacea for relentless time and labor demands, dedicated farmers in both communities continue to work diligently in these projects in hopes of making organic production a possibility for their heavily burdened neighbors.

Confronting the knowledge-dependence treadmill

In addition to substantial investments of time and labor, chemical-free farming also depends on the control and application of farming knowledge. Many farmers derive their knowledge of cultivation—especially agrochemical application—from the advice of industry "experts," often agrochemical companies or distributors who profit from their use. Chapter Two showed in detail how farmers' lack of understanding of safe chemical applications and dosages and inability to resolve problems in the field without using chemicals contribute to greater pesticide use and poisonings. These problems are symptoms of the broader knowledge-dependence treadmill faced by farmers in both the coffee and fresh vegetable commodity chains.

In the case of Bella Vista, nearly all residents were former employees of conventional coffee plantations where they were taught to grow coffee only with heavy applications of chemicals. For this reason, learning to grow coffee without chemical inputs was frustrating for many farmers, who found it more reliable and familiar to continue using conventional coffee-growing techniques using heavy chemical applications.

We observed similar processes of knowledge dependence in San Carlos, where farming information came almost exclusively from agrochemical retailers. Because many farmers, such as Don Josue, first learned about cultivation techniques by working on conventional farms, they only knew to apply more agrochemicals and integrate new, more potent products when problems arose in the field. For Don Josue, the only way to determine which chemicals to use was to inquire of the vendors. With a vested interest in selling more products, these sellers counsel that more is always better. As a woman new to farming in a community described by our informants as highly *machista*, Doña Josefina found herself in a similar situation. She felt too intimidated and inexperienced to question the technical farming knowledge offered to her by almost exclusively male chemical retailers.

Compounding these knowledge dynamics is the intense competition in such saturated agricultural markets as those in Guatemala, which has fostered an atmosphere of egoism and individualism. Rather than collaborate and share their experiences with effective pest-avoidance techniques or bountiful harvests, farmers tend to withhold from one another the lessons they learn through their own successful farming practices, even going so far as to transport chemicals in mismarked bottles in an effort to disguise their intentions from their neighbors.

Programs aiming to reduce agrochemical dependence among small farmers must replace chemical retailers and vendors as the primary sources of agricultural information and techniques at the local level. Farmer education can and does contribute to breaking knowledge dependence. However, to begin developing effective alternatives to hazardous chemical use, public health programs must facilitate a re-embedding of agricultural production techniques in the experience-based knowledge of farmers and farmer groups. Programs promoting reduced-chemical agriculture must go beyond simplistic, top-down transfers of knowledge of sustainable farming practices from agriculture and public health professionals to farmers. They must instead start by building information-sharing networks in which farmers themselves feel comfortable developing and maintaining a shared body of knowledge by communicating their experiences concerning different farming techniques.

In the examples discussed in this book, building a collective farmer enterprise and business venture helped to reduce competitive pressures that previously had pitted farmers against one another. Participation in a joint venture offered these farmers an incentive for sharing information about cultivation techniques. Many felt invested in the success of the enterprise and the benefits it brought to them and their communities. Creating such an avenue for the sharing of experiences—not just feeding farmers external knowledge but facilitating the creating of social networks and social institutions for generating and sharing knowledge— can be especially important for programs promoting farmer transitions to agroecology or other agricultural techniques based in local ecological processes. To do so, programs must integrate participatory elements such as collaborative development of agricultural techniques and hands-on group experimentation in test plots.

Critically, facilitating farmer information-sharing requires a deep understanding of group dynamics at the local level. Designers of public health and agrarian development projects must rely heavily on in-depth research concerning the goals and incentives that motivate farmers to participate in local groups and share information. Development organizations that understand local conditions and needs can generate farmer interest in a given initiative or program more effectively. At the same time, the farmers themselves must play the central role of constructing these information-sharing networks and disseminating successful agricultural practices that are based on their own experiments in agriculture.

In both Bella Vista and San Carlos, breaking from knowledge dependence on agrochemical experts or previously learned conventional farming techniques was truly a community effort, led, in large part, by groups of farmers themselves. In many ways paralleling what Eric Holt-Giménez (2006) describes as Campesino Pedagogy, rural community members worked with development and public health professionals to form collaborative farmer groups where previously none existed. Through highly interactive, hands-on workshops and meetings, farmers, as a group, began to analyze the problems that they had experienced with converting to chemical-free agriculture. A group-led analysis of problems developed into experimentation with alternatives in the field. Now, as working solutions are developed, farmers disseminate this experience-based knowledge to others in meetings of producer institutions like POSC or the Organic Group of Bella Vista. Through these collaborative endeavors and with the support of outside NGOs or other institutions, group composting projects, vermicultures, or new approaches to marketing agricultural goods are developed. In this way, farmers in Bella Vista and San Carlos have lightened the pressures of the knowledge-dependence treadmill and have begun to reclaim knowledge of agricultural processes, allowing them to minimize or eliminate the need for potentially toxic agrochemicals in farming.

For the Bella Vista and San Carlos farmers, the formation of these institutions was pivotal in developing practical farming solutions that address the public health threats introduced by agrochemical use. Beyond knowledge sharing, the Organic Group of Bella Vista retained many of its members due to the support it provided in farming materials, credits, and education. Even as conventional coffee market prices approached prevailing prices in the organic markets, many farmers find the benefits of collaboration and the resulting social capital (Coleman 1988) to be reason enough to continue farming organically (Bacon 2005 and Bray et al. 2002 report similar findings among coffee cooperatives in Mexico and Nicaragua). In an environment of high competition, egoism, and *machismo*, collaboration by the San Carlos vegetable farmers of POSC led from the development of alternative farming techniques to the formation of a fledgling microenterprise. Translating this social capital into human capital with a degree of modest success, many POSC farmers have become expert promoters of agroecology, customer service personnel, and product developers in a local organic food system. They have created a small but growing base of urban consumers in Quetzaltenango who are interested in purchasing chemical-free products. With the help of NGO partners, they have converted this demand into economic incentives for members to continue working to rid themselves of agrochemical use in farming. As a result, POSC farmers in San Carlos have opened a new avenue for produce sales that, once developed, has the potential to allow them to preserve their own and their communities' health, while still participating in the commercial cultivation of fresh vegetables.

Confronting the quality-preference treadmill

In this book, we have provided two distinct examples of market development for specialty agricultural products, one global and one local. In these cases, the choice of marketing strategy depended on local resources, capabilities, infrastructural development, export crop histories, and commodity chain characteristics. Public health and agricultural development programs had a strong role in breaking the cycle of quality preference. By helping to develop specialty products like Organic and Fair-Trade Certified coffees or a mixed bag of eco-vegetables for local distribution, collaborations between public health or development specialists and farmer groups have made great strides in developing new markets that sustain chemical-free agriculture. Again, the message is clear: programs that seek to promote reduced-chemical agriculture must go beyond the one-way promotion of organic practices and technologies to farmers and farmer groups. The adoption and development of these agricultural techniques by farmers will be short-lived in the absence of adequate reinforcement and input from the farmers themselves. Programs to address chemical use by small farmers must consider sustainable agricultural production and market development as two halves of the same whole. Both must be secured in order to address overuse of toxic agrochemicals. Following this approach, public health and agrarian development programs can begin to address the economic roots of agrochemical use and the resulting threats to public health by developing alternative markets for farmers interested in reducing hazardous chemical use to protect themselves and their communities.

In the cases we have discussed, the role of context-based knowledge uncovered through long-term collaboration with farmers and ethnographic research was central to success. In addition, a program's ability to maximize options available to farmers at the local level, while also developing their specific capabilities to meet market standards, is crucial and is heavily influenced by the context-specific factors that are best uncovered through direct ethnographic research. Specifically, the ability of farmers and farmer groups to sustain markets for low-chemical agricultural products is dependent on a host of factors, including local human capital, available infrastructures for delivering products to distant markets, and the ability to cater to specific notions of quality held by consumers. Here, development initiatives can support alternative commodity chains that reward farmers for practicing reduced-chemical agriculture while meeting consumer demands on product quality. Such alternative commodity chains must be context-specific, tailored to farmer needs and consumer preferences, and guided by insights best uncovered through ethnographic research on the needs of all involved stakeholders.

Small farmers in Guatemala, like many across the developing world, have become inextricably integrated into the production of agricultural commodities on terms dictated by the variety of players in the global market. In many cases, the requirements of purchasers lead to specific demands on production that give rise to seemingly intractable threats to public health. Though they do not offer silver-bullet solutions to the hazards of agrochemical use, the two examples in this book demonstrate how farmer-run institutions of collaboration can result in the generation of alternatives to chemically-intense farming that make use of local resources and capabilities. More generally, the farmers in Bella Vista and San Carlos have shown that individuals in the developing world are not passive subjects of global processes but are instead active shapers of their own livelihoods and community well-being.

A counter-momentum is growing in response to the treadmills that drive agrochemical poisonings in developing countries. Active groups of agricultural commodity producers are assembling, collaborating, and sharing stories and experiences of both success and setback in eliminating the threats to family and community health posed by agrochemicals. Though these groups still have significant barriers to overcome in order to fully achieve their goals, participating members are charting a clearer path toward a workable household livelihood strategy that includes both agriculture pursuits and the health security of their families and neighbors. In doing so, they demonstrate an unshakable and contagious hope that they will succeed in breaking the momentum of the treadmills that drive agrochemical related health threats in their communities. While the long-term objective of chemical-free agricultural production may still lie in the distant future, the stories shared in this book demonstrate ways in which farmers can take measured and practical steps to effect change that is having impacts both within their communities and throughout the chains connecting them to the global market. A young member of Bella Vista's Organic Group concludes our story :

> There are distinct manners of thinking, and those who follow what is called organic, I think, it is because they have noticed the contamina-

tion in recent years. So from here they will not persist in this contamination. So it is necessary to work a little, do what we can to help the environment a little, that has given us so much and we continue killing it with so many chemical products. So, I think that is the reason why some of us are still working in what is organic production.... My goals are, for example, for my children, is to give them an education, too. Yes. Give them as much of an education as they want. As far as the community, in terms of working, perhaps [my goal is] that everyone else will come to understand what is called organic work. Maybe it's not for us, but for our children. There is already enough contamination and it is no longer possible to continue. So, [my goal is] that everyone will want to work [organic] and in this way help a little to maintain the community or maybe clean it a little. Yes, that would be my goal, to keep the community clean.

References

Aiello, Allison E. and Elaine L. Larson
    2002   What Is the Evidence for a Causal Link between Hygiene and Infections? *Lancet Infectious Diseases* 2:103–110.

Altieri, Miguel A.
    1995   *Agroecology: The Science of Sustainable Agriculture.* Boulder, CO: Westview Press.

Amigos de La Tierra, Quetzaltenango (ATQ)
    2006   Diagnóstico del Cantón Comunidad de los Pinos. M.A. thesis, Division de Ciencia y Technología, Universidad de San Carlos de Guatemala.
    2002   Diagnóstico General del Cantón Comunidad de las Nubes, Valle de San Carlos, Municipio de Quetzaltenango, Departamento de Quetzaltenango. M.A. thesis, División de Ciencia y Tecnología, Universidad de San Carlos de Guatemala.
    2001a   Diagnóstico General del Cantón Comunidad del Río, Municipio de Quetzaltenango, Departamento de Quetzaltenango. División de Ciencia y Tecnología, Universidad de San Carlos de Guatemala.
    2001b   Diagnóstico del Cantón Comunidad de la Loma del Valle de San Carlos, Quetzaltenango. M.A. thesis. División de Ciencia y Tecnología, Universidad de San Carlos de Guatemala.

Arbona, Sonia I.
    1998   Commercial Agriculture and Agrochemicals in Almolonga, Guatemala. *Geographical Review* 88:47–63.

Bacon, Christopher M.
    2005   Confronting the Coffee Crisis: Can Fair Trade, Organic, and Specialty Coffees Reduce Small-Scale Farmer Vulnerability in Northern Nicaragua? *World Development* 33(3):497–511.

Bair, Jennifer
    2005   Global Capitalism and Commodity Chains: Looking Back, Going Forward. *Competition and Change* 9(2):153–180.

Barrett, Bruce
    1995   Commentary: Plants, Pesticides and Production in Guatemala: Nutrition, Health and Nontraditional Agriculture. *Ecology of Food and Nutrition* 33:293–309.

Bazylewicz-Walczak, B., W. Majczakowa, and M. Szymczak
    1999   Behavioral Effects of Occupational Exposure to Organophosphorous Pesticides in Female Greenhouse Planting Workers. *Neurotoxicology* 20(5):819–826.

Beck, Ulrich
    1992   *Risk Society: Towards a New Modernity.* London: SAGE Publications.

Beckett, Megan and Anne R. Pebley
    2003   Ethnicity, Language, and Economic Well-Being in Rural Guatemala. *Rural Sociology* 68:434-458.

Berger, Susan
    1992   *Political and Agrarian Development in Guatemala.* Boulder, CO: Westview Press.

Bhatt, M. H., M. A. Elias, and A. K. Mankodi
  1999   Acute and Reversible Parkinsonism Due to Organophosphate Pesticide Intoxication:
          Five Cases. *Neurology* 52:1467–1471.
Bolognesi, Claudia
  2003   Genotoxicity of Pesticides: A Review of Human Biomonitoring Studies. *Mutation Re-
          search* 543:251–272.
Bowser, Diana M. and Ajay Mahal
  2010   Guatemala: The Economic Burden of Illness and Health System Implications. *Health
          Policy* 100:159–166.
Bray, David Barton, Jose Luis Plaza Sanchez, and Ellen Contreras Murphy
  2002   Social Dimensions of Organic Coffee Production in Mexico: Lessons for Eco-Labeling
          Initiatives. *Society and Natural Resources* 15:429–446.
Breman, Anna and Carolyn Shelton
  2007   Structural Adjustment Programs and Health. In *Globalization and Health,* I. Kawachi
          and S. Wamala, eds. 219–233. New York: Oxford University Press.
Britnell, George E.
  1958   Problemas del Cambio Económico y Social en Guatemala. In *Economía de Guatemala.
          Seminario de Integración Social Guatemalteca.* 47–77. Guatemala City: Editorial del
          Ministerio de Educación Pública.
Brockett, Charles D.
  1998   *Land, Power, and Poverty: Agrarian Transformation and Political Conflict in Central
          America (2nd Edition).* Boulder, CO: Westview Press.
Buccini, John
  2004   *The Global Pursuit of the Sound Management of Chemicals.* Washington DC: The Inter-
          national Bank for Reconstruction and Development/The World Bank.
Calo, Muriel and Timothy A. Wise
  2005   *Revaluing Peasant Coffee Production.* Medford, MA: Global Development and Environ-
          ment Institute, Tufts University.
Calvert, Geoffrey M., Louise N. Mehler, Rachel Rosales, Lynden Baum, Catherine Thomsen, Dorilee
Male, Omar Shafey, Rupali Das, Michelle Lackovic, and Ernest Arvizu
  2003   Acute Pesticide-Related Illnesses among Working Youths, 1988–1999. *American Journal
          of Public Health* 93(4):605–610.
Carmack, Robert
  1988   *Harvest of Violence: Maya Indians and the Guatemalan Crisis.* Norman, OK: University
          of Oklahoma Press.
Castillejos, Teresa, Elizabeth Baer, and Bambi Semroc
  2010   "Guatemala Field Survey Report." Technical Report. Arlington, VA: Conservation Inter-
          national.
Chambers, Robert
  2007   "From PRA to PLA and Pluralism: Practice and Theory." IDS Working Paper 286. Brigh-
          ton: Institute of Development Studies at the University of Sussex.
Chancellor, A. M., J. M. Slattery, H. Fraser, and C. P. Warlow
  1993   Risk Factors for Motor Neuron Disease—A Case-Control Study Based on Patients from
          the Scottish Motor Neuron Disease Register. *Journal of Neurology, Neurosurgery, and
          Psychiatry with Practical Neurology* 56:1200–1206.
Chenery, Hollis
  1961   Comparative Advantage and Development Policy. *American Economic Review* 51(1):18–
          51.
Cochrane, Willard W.
  1958   *Farm Prices: Myth and Reality.* St. Paul: University of Minnesota Press.
Cole, Donald C., Fernando Carpio, Jim Julian, Ninfa Leon, Ramona Carbotte,
and Hipatia De Almeida
  1997   Neurobehavioral Outcomes among Farm and Nonfarm Rural Ecuadorians. *Neurotoxi-
          cology and Teratology* 19(4):277–286.

Coleman, James S.
　　1988　　Social Capital in the Creation of Human Capital, *American Journal of Sociology* 94
　　　　　　Supplement: S95–S120.
Collier, Paul and Jan Willem Gunning
　　1999　　The IMF's role in structural adjustment. *The Economic Journal* 109:634–651.
Comision Internacional contra la Impunidad en Guatemala (CICIG)
　　n.d.　　Mandato: Acuerdo de creacion de la CICIG
Connan, C.
　　1996　　*Health Care Providers' Knowledge of Pesticide Related Illness and Treatment.* Seattle, WA:
　　　　　　University of Washington.
Conroy, Michael E., Douglas L. Murray, and Peter M. Rosset
　　1996　　*A Cautionary Tale; Failed U.S. Development Policy in Central America.* Boulder, CO:
　　　　　　Lynne Rienner Publishers, Inc.
Corriols Molina, Marianela
　　2009　　Acute Pesticide Poisonings in Nicaragua: Underreporting, Incidence and Determinants.
　　　　　　Ph.D. thesis, Department of Public Health Sciences, Division of Occupational and Envi-
　　　　　　ronmental Medicine, Stockholm, Sweden: Karolinska Institutet.
Curtis, K. M., D. A. Savitz, C. R. Weeinberg, and T. E. Arbuckle
　　1999　　The Effect of Pesticide Exposure on Time to Pregnancy. *Epidemiology* 10(2):112–117.
Daniell, William, Scott Barnhart, Paul Demers, Lucio G. Costa, David L. Eaton, Mary Miller, and
Linda Rosenstock
　　1992　　Neuropsychological Performance among Agricultural Pesticide Applicators. *Environ-
　　　　　　mental Research* 59(1):217–228.
Daniels, Julie L., Andrew F. Olshan, and David A. Savitz
　　1997　　Pesticides and Childhood Cancers. *Environmental Health Perspectives* 105(10):1068–
　　　　　　1077.
De Janvry, Alain
　　1972　　Optimal Levels of Fertilization Under Risk: The Potential for Corn and Wheat Fertiliza-
　　　　　　tion Under Alternative Price Policies in Argentina. *American Journal of Agricultural
　　　　　　Economics* 54(1):1–10.
DeWalt, Darren A., Nancy D. Berkman, Stacey Sheridan, Kathleen N. Lohr, and Michael P. Pignone
　　2004　　Literacy and Health Outcomes: A Systematic Review of the Literature. *Journal of General
　　　　　　Internal Medicine* 19:1228–1239.
Dich, Jan, Shelia Hoar Zahm, Annika Hanberg, and Hans-Olov Adami
　　1997　　Pesticides and Cancer. *Cancer Causes and Control* 8:420–443.
Dick R., K. Steenland, E. Krieg, and C. Hines
　　2001　　Evaluation of Acute Sensory-Motor Effects and Test Sensitivity using Termiticide Work-
　　　　　　ers Exposed to Chlorpyrifos. *Neurotoxicology and Teratology* 23:381–393.
Dolan, C. and J. Humphrey
　　2000　　Governance and Trade in Fresh Vegetables: The Impact of UK Supermarkets on the
　　　　　　African Horticulture Industry. *Journal of Development Studies* 37(2):147–176.
Dollar, David and Jakob Svensson
　　2000　　What Explains the Success or Failure of Structural Adjustment Programmes? *The Eco-
　　　　　　nomic Journal* 110:894–917.
Dosemeci, Mustafa, Robert N. Hoover, Aaron Blair, Larry W. Figgs, Susan Devesa, Dan Grauman,
and Joseph F. Fraumeni Jr.
　　1994　　Farming and Prostate Cancer among African–Americans in the Southeastern United
　　　　　　States (Brief communication). *Journal of the National Cancer Institute* 86(22):1718–9.
Dowdall, Courtney
　　2012　　Small Farmer Market Knowledge and Specialty Coffee Commodity Chains in Western
　　　　　　Highlands Guatemala. Ph.D. dissertation, Department of Global and Sociocultural Stud-
　　　　　　ies, Miami, FL: Florida International University.
Ecobichon, Donald J.
　　2001　　Toxic Effects of Pesticides. In Casarett and Doull's *Toxicology: The Basic Science of Poi-
　　　　　　sons, 6th Edition.* Curtis D. Klaassen. ed. 763–811. New York: McGraw-Hill.

The Economist
   2009   Malnutrition in Guatemala: A National Shame. *The Economist*, August 27.
Ehlers, Tracy Bachrach
   2000   *Silent Looms: Women and Production in a Guatemalan Town. 2nd Edition.* Austin, TX: University of Texas Press.
Ellis, Frank
   1993   *Peasant Economics: Farm Households and Agrarian Development, 2nd Edition,* Cambridge, UK: Cambridge University Press.
Eng, Eugenia, John Briscoe, and Anne Cunningham
   1990   Participation Effect from Water Projects on EPI. *Social Science & Medicine* 30(12): 1349–1358.
Engel, Lawrence S., Matthew C. Keifer, Harvey Checkoway, Lawrence R. Robinson, and Thomas L. Vaughan
   1998   Neurophysiological Function in Farm Workers Exposed to Organophosphate Pesticides. *Archives of Environmental Health* 53(1):7–14.
Environmental Protection Agency (EPA)
   2012   In Case of Pesticide Poisoning. http://www.epa.gov/oppfead1/safety/incaseof.htm, accessed February 25, 2013.
Eswaran, Mukesh and Ashok Kotwal
   1989   Credit as Insurance in Agrarian Economies. *Journal of Development Economics* 31(1):37–53.
Evans, B. E., L. Haller, and G. Hutton
   2004   Closing the Sanitation Gap: The Case for Better Public Funding of Sanitation and Hygiene Report. Paris: OECD.
Farahat, T. M., G. M. Abdelrasoul, M. M. Amr, M. M. Shebl, F. M. Farahat, and W. K. Anger
   2003   Neurobehavioral Effects among Workers Occupationally Exposed to Organophosphorous Pesticides. *Occupational & Environmental Medicine* 60(4):279–286.
Fares, Jean and Dhushyanth Raju
   2007   Child Labor across the Developing World: Patterns and Correlations. World Bank Policy Research Working Paper, 4119: World Bank. The World Region.
Fenske, R.A.
   1997   Pesticide Exposure Assessment of Workers and Their Families. *Occupational Medicine* 12:221–237.
Fernando, Ravindra, D. G. Harendra De Silva, and T. S. D. Amarasena
   1990   An Unusual Case of Fatal Accidental Paraquat Poisoning. *Forensic Science International* 44(1):23–26.
Fieten, Karin B., Hans Kromhout, Dick Heederik, and Berna van Wendel de Joode
   2009   Pesticide Exposure and Respiratory Health of Indigenous Women in Costa Rica. *American Journal of Epidemiology* 169(12):1500–1506.
Filmer, Deon, Jeffrey S. Hammer, and Land H. Pritchett
   2000   Weak Links in the Chain: A Diagnosis of Health Policy in Poor Countries. *The World Bank Research Observer* 15(2):199–224.
Fischer, Edward F. and Peter Benson
   2006   *Broccoli and Desire: Global Connections and Maya Struggles in Postwar Guatemala.* Stanford, CA: Stanford University Press.
Fletcher, Lehman B.
   1970   Guatemala's Economic Development: The Role of Agriculture. Ames, IA: Iowa State University Press.
Food and Agriculture Organization (FAO) of the United Nations
   2002   International Code of Conduct on the Distribution and Use of Pesticides. http://www.fao.org/agriculture/crops/core-themes/theme/pests/code/en/, accessed February 20, 2013.
Fridell, Gavin
   2007   *Fair Trade Coffee: The Prospects and Pitfalls of Market-Driven Social Justice.* Toronto: University of Toronto Press.

Gereffi, Gary
 1994 The Organization of Buyer-Driven Global Commodity Chains: How U.S. Retailers Shape
  Overseas Production Networks. In *Commodity Chains and Global Capitalism*, Gary
  Gereffi and Miguel Korzeniewicz, eds. 95–122. Westport, CT: Praeger.
Gereffi, Gary, John Humphrey, and Timothy Sturgeon
 2005 The Governance of Global Value Chains. *Review of International Political Economy*
  12(1):78–104.
Giddens, Anthony
 1990 *The Consequences of Modernity.* Stanford, CA: Stanford University Press.
Gliessman, Stephen R.
 1998 *Agroecology: Ecological Processes in Sustainable Agriculture.* Chelsea, MI: Ann Arbor
  Press.
Goldín, Liliana
 2009 *Global Maya: Work and Ideology in Rural Guatemala.* Tucson: The University of Arizona
  Press.
Goldman, Noreen, Anne R. Pebley, and Megan Beckett
 2001 Diffusion of Ideas about Personal Hygiene and Contamination in Poor Countries: Evi-
  dence from Guatemala. *Social Science and Medicine* 52:53–69.
Goldman, Noreen, Anne R. Pebley, and Michele Gragnolati
 2000 Choices about Treatment for ARI and Diarrhea in Rural Guatemala. On-line Working
  Paper Series. Los Angeles: California Center for Population Research.
Gomes J., O. L. Lloyd, and D. M. Revitt
 1999 The Influence of Personal Protection, Environmental Hygiene and Exposure to Pesticides on the Health of Immigrant Farm Workers in a Desert Country. *International
  Archives of Occupational and Environmental Health* 72:40–45.
Gragnolati, Michele and Alessandra Marini
 2003 Health and Poverty in Guatemala. Policy Research Working Paper 2966. The World
  Bank. World Bank, Latin American and Caribbean Sector, Washington, D.C.
Granieri, E., M. Carreras, and R. Tola
 1988 Motor Neuron Disease in the Province of Ferrara, Italy, in 1964–1982. *Neurology*
  38:1604–1608.
Gresser, Charis, and Sophia Tickell
 2002 *Mugged: Poverty in your Coffee Cup.* Oxford: Oxfam International.
Grübler, Arnulf
 2003 *Technology and Global Change.* Cambridge, UK: Cambridge University Press.
Guidotti, Tee L. and Benjamin A. Gitterman
 2007 Global Pediatric Environmental Health. *Pediatric Clinics of North America* 54(2):335–
  350.
Gupta, Sanjeev, Marijn Verhoeven, and Erwin R. Tiongson
 2002 The Effectiveness of Government Spending on Education and Health Care in Developing Economies. *European Journal of Political Economy* 18:717–737.
Hamilton, Sara and Edward Fischer
 2005 Maya Farmers and Export Agriculture in Highland Guatemala: Implications for Development and Labor Relations. *Latin American Perspectives* 32(5):33–58.
 2003 Non-Traditional Agricultural Exports in Highland Guatemala: Understandings of Risk
  and Perceptions of Change. *Latin American Research Review* 38(3):82–110.
Hanke, Wojciech and Joanna Jurewicz
 2004 The Risk of Adverse Reproductive and Developmental Disorders due to Occupational
  Pesticide Exposure: An Overview of Current Epidemiological Evidence. *International
  Journal of Occupational and Environmental Health* 17(2):223–243.
Harari, Raul, Francesco Forastiere, and Olav Axelson
 1997 Unacceptable "Occupational" Exposure to Toxic Agents among Children in Ecuador.
  American Journal of Industrial Medicine 32:185–189.

Harris, Jessica and Andrew McCartor
    2011   The World's Worst Toxic Pollution Problems Report; The Top Ten of the Toxic Twenty.
            Technical Report 2011. New York: Blacksmith Institute.
Hines, Cynthia J., James A. Deddens, Samuel P. Tucker, and Richard W. Hornung
    2001   Distributions and Determinants of Pre-Emergent Herbicide Exposures Among Custom
            Applicators. *The Annals of Occupational Hygiene* 45:227–239.
Hogstedt, Christer, David H. Wegman, and Tord Kjellstrom
    2007   The Consequences of Economic Globalization on Working Conditions, Labor Relations,
            and Worker's Health. In *Globalization and Health,* Ichiro Kawachi and Sarah Wamala,
            eds. 138–157. New York: Oxford University Press.
Holt-Giménez, Eric
    2006   *Campesino a Campesino: Voices from Latin America's Farmer to Farmer Movement for
            Sustainable Agriculture.* Oakland, CA: Food First Books.
Hurst, Peter
    1999   Safe Use in Guatemala—Are Industry Projects Effective? *Pesticide News* 43:8–9.
International Coffee Organization (ICO)
    n.d. a All Exporting Countries Prices Paid to Growers (in current terms) Annual averages:2000
            to 2009. http://www.ico.org/historical/2000-09/PDF/PricestoGrowers.pdf, accessed
            February 25, 2013.
    n.d. b Prices Paid to Growers in Current Terms, Calendar year average 1975 to 1989. http://
            www.ico.org/historical/1990-99/PDF/PricestoGrowers90-99.pdf, accessed February 25,
            2013.
Israel, Barbara A., Amy J. Schulz, Edith A. Parker, and Adam B. Becker
    1998   Review of Community-Based Research: Assessing Partnership Approaches to Improve
            Public Health. *Annual Review of Public Health* 19:173–202.
Jabloniká, Angelika, Helena Poláková, Jarmila Karelová, and Mária Vargová
    1989   Analysis of Chromosome Aberrations and Sister-Chromatid Exchanges in Peripheral
            Blood Lymphocytes of Workers with Occupational Exposure to the Mancozeb contain-
            ing Fungicide Novozir Mn80. *Mutation Research/Genetic Toxicology* 224(2):143–146.
Jaffee, Daniel
    2007   *Brewing Justice: Fair Trade Coffee, Sustainability, and Survival.* Berkeley: University of
            California Press.
Jeyaratnam, J.
    1990   Acute Pesticide Poisoning: A Major Global Health Problem. *World Health Statistics
            Quarterly* 43(3):139–144.
Kamel, Freya and Jane A. Hoppin
    2004   Association of Pesticide Exposure with Neurologic Dysfunction and Disease. *Environ-
            mental Health Perspectives* 112(9):950–958.
Kamel, Freya, Andrew S. Rowland, Lawrence P. Park, W. Kent Anger, Donna D. Baird, Beth C.
Gladen, Tirso Moreno, Lillian Stallone, and Dale P. Sandler
    2003   Neurobehavioral Performance and Work Experience in Florida Farmworkers. *Environ-
            mental Health Perspectives* 111(14):1765–1772.
Kaplinsky, Raphael
    2004   Competitions Policy and the Global Coffee and Cocoa Value Chains. Geneva: Paper
            Prepared for the United Nations Conference for Trade and Development (UNCTAD).
Kegley, S. E., B. R. Hill, S. Orme, and A. H. Choi
    2010   *PAN Pesticide Database: Paraquat dichloride. San Francisco:* Electronic document.
            Pesticide Action Network. http://www.pesticideinfo.org/Detail_Chemical.jsp?Rec_
            Id=PC33358, accessed February 28, 2013.
Keifer, M. and R. Mahurin
    1997   Chronic Neurologic Effects of Pesticide Overexposure. *Occupational Medicine* 12:291–
            304.

Kolilekas, L., E. Ghizopoulou, S. Retsou, S. Kourelea, and C. Hadjistavrou
    2006   Severe Paraquat Poisoning. A Long-Term Survivor. *Respiratory Medicine Extra* 2(2):67–70.

Konefal, Jason, Carmen Bain, Michael Mascarenhaus, and Lawrence Busch
    2007   Supermarkets and Supply Chains in North America. In *Supermarkets and Agri-Food Supply Chains: Transformations in the Production and Consumption of Foods,* David Burch and Geofrrey Lawrence, eds. 268–288. Cheltenham, UK: Edward Elgar Publishing Limited.

Korsak, R.J. and M.M. Sato
    1977   Effects of Organophosphate Pesticides Chronic Exposure on the Central Nervous System. *Clinical Toxicology* 11:83–95.

Kourakis, A., M. Mouratidou, G. Kokkinos, A. Barbouti, A. Kotsis, D. Mourelatos, and J. Dozi-Vassiliades
    1992   Frequencies of Chromosomal Aberrations in Pesticide Sprayers Working in Plastic Green Houses. *Mutation Research* 279:145–148.

Levy, Barry S. and Victor W. Sidel
    2003   War and Public Health in the Twenty-First Century. *New England Journal of Public Policy* 19(1):167–178.

Lewis, Maureen
    2006   Governance and Corruption in Public Health Care Systems. Working Paper, 78. Washington, D.C.: Center for Global Development.

London, Leslie, Sylvie de Grosbois, Catharina Wesseling, Sophia Kisting, Hanna Andrea Rother, and Donna Mergler
    2002   Pesticide Usage and Health Consequences for Women in Developing Countries: Out of Sight, Out of Mind? *International Journal of Occupational Environmental Health* 8:26–59.

London, Leslie and Jonathan E. Myers
    1998   Use of a Crop and Job Specific Exposure Matrix for Retrospective Assessment of Long-Term Exposure in Studies of Chronic Neurotoxic Effects of Agrichemicals. *Occupational & Environmental Medicine* 55:194–201.

London, L., J. E. Myers, V. Nell, T. Taylor, and M. L. Thompson
    1997   An Investigation into Neurologic and Neurobehavioral Effects of Long-Term Agrichemical Use among Deciduous Fruit Farm Workers in the Western Cape, South Africa. *Environmental Research* 73(1–2):132–145.

London, Leslie, Victor Nell, Mary-Lou Thompson, and Jonathan E. Myers
    1998   Effects of Long-Term Organophosphate Exposures on Neurological Symptoms, Vibration Sense and Tremor among South African Farm Workers. *Scandinavian Journal of Work and Environmental Health* 24:18–29.

Lyon, Sarah
    2009   What Good Will Two More Trees Do?' The Political Economy of Sustainable Coffee Certification, Local Livelihoods and Identities. *Landscape Research* 34(2)223–240.

Lyons, G.
    1999   Pesticides Posing Hazards to Reproduction. http://www.pan-k.org/pestnews/Actives/endocrin.htm, accessed February 20, 2013.

Maizlish, N., M. Schenker, C. Weisskoph, J. Seiber, and S. Samuels
    1987   A Behavioral Evaluation of Pest Control Workers with Short-Term, Low-Level Exposure to the Organophosphate Diazinon. *American Journal of Industrial Medicine* 12:153–172.

Makinen, M., H. Waters, M. Rauch, N. Almagambetova, R. Bitran, L. Gilson, D. McIntyre, S. Pannarunothai, A. L. Prieto, G. Ubilla, and S. Ram
    2000   Inequalities in Health Care Use and Expenditures: Empirical Data from Eight Developing Countries in Transition. *Bulletin of the World Health Organization* 78:55–65.

Matson, P. A., W. J. Parton, A. G. Power, and M. J. Swift
    1997   Agricultural Intensification and Ecosystem Properties. *Science* 277(5325):504–509.

Mathews, Rahel, Chen Reis, and Vincent Iacopino
    2003   Child Labor: A Matter of Health and Human Rights. *Journal of Ambulatory Care Management* 26(2):181–182.
Matthew, G. A.
    2008   Attitudes and Behaviours Regarding Use of Crop Protection Products—A Survey of More than 8500 Smallholders in 26 Countries. *Crop Protection* 27:834–846.
May, Rachel
    2001   *Terror in the Countryside: Campesino Response to Political Violence in Guatemala, 1954–1985.* Athens, OH: Ohio University Press.
Maya, Diego
    2010   CICIG investigation leads to arrest of former public officials. http://infosurhoy.com/cocoon/saii/xhtml/en_GB/features/saii/features/society/2010/08/19/feature-02, accessed August 19, 2013.
McCauley, Linda A., W. Kent Anger, Matthew Keifer, Rick Langley, Mark G. Robson, and Diane Rohlman
    2006   Studying Health Outcomes in Farmworker Populations Exposed to Pesticides. *Environmental Health Perspectives* 114(6):953–960.
McTaggart, J. and W. Heller
    2005   Forces of Change. *Progressive Grocer* 84(6):48–60.
Minority Rights Group International
    2009   State of the World's Minorities and Indigenous Peoples 2009—Guatemala. http://www.unhcr.org/refworld/topic,463af2212,469f2e812,4a66d9b550,0.html, accessed February 24, 2013.
Miranda, Jamilette, Rob McConnell, Edgar Delgado, Ricardo Cuadra, Matthew Keifer, Catharina Wesseling, Edmundo Torres, and Ingvar Lundberg
    2002   Tactile Vibration Thresholds after Acute Poisonings with Organophosphate Insecticides. *International Journal of Occupational and Environmental Health* 8(3):212–219.
Montgomery, Maggie A. and Menachem Elimelech
    2007   Water and Sanitation in Developing Countries: Including Health in the Equation. *Environmental Science & Technology* 16–24.
Mull, Diane L. and Steven R. Kirkhorn
    2005   Child Labor in Ghana Cocoa Production: Focus upon Agricultural Tasks, Ergonomic Exposures, and Associated Injuries and Illnesses. *Public Health Reports* 120(6):649–656.
Murdoch, Jonathan and M. Miele
    1999   "Back to Nature": Changing "Worlds of Production" in the Food Sector. *Sociologia Ruralis* 39(4):465–483.
Murray, Douglas and Peter Leigh Taylor
    2000   Claim No Easy Victories: Evaluating the Pesticide Industry's Global Safe Use Campaign. *World Development* 28(10):1735–1749.
Murray, Douglas, Catharina Wesseling, Matthew Keifer, Marianela Corriols, and Samuel Henao
    2002   Surveillance of Pesticide-Related Illness in the Developing World: Putting the Data to Work. *International Journal of Occupational Health* 8(3):243–248.
Mutersbaugh, Tad
    2002   The Number is the Beast: A Political Economy of Organic-Coffee Certification and Producer Unionism. *Environment and Planning* A 34(7):1165–1184.
National Environmental Education and Training Foundation
    2002   *National Strategies for Health Care Providers: Pesticides Initiative Implementation Plan.* Washington, DC: National Environmental Education and Training Foundation.
Nehez, M., P. Boros, A. Ferke, J. Mohos, M. Palotas, G. Vetro, M. Zimanyl, and I. Desi
    1988   Cytogenetic Examination of People Working With Agrochemicals in the Southern Region of Hungary. *Regulatory Toxicology and Pharmacology* 8(1):37–44.
New York Times Health Guide
    n.d.   Insecticide Poisoning. http://health.nytimes.com/health/guides/poison/insecticide/overview.html, accessed February 25, 2013.

Ohayo-Mitoko, G. J., H. Kromhout, J. M. Simwa, J. S. Boleij, and D. Heederik
  2000   Self Reported Symptoms and Inhibition of Acetylcholinesterase Activity among Kenyan
          Agricultural Workers. *Journal of Occupational and Environmental Medicine* 57:195–200.
Organisation for Economic Co-operation and Development (OECD)
  2011   Public social spending. In *Society at a Glance 2011: OECD Social Indicators*, 74–75.
          OECD Publishing.
Padmavathi, P., P. A. Prabhavathi, and P. P. Reddy
  2000   Frequencies of SCEs in Peripheral Blood Lymphocytes of Pesticide Workers. *Bulletin of
          Environmental Contamination and Toxicology* 64:155–160.
Padungtod, Chantana, Tianhua Niu, Zhaoxi Wang, David A. Savitz, David C. Cristiani,
Louise M. Ryan, and Xiping Xu
  1999   Paraoxonase Polymorphism and its Effect on Male Reproductive Outcomes among Chi-
          nese Pesticide Factory Workers. *American Journal of Industrial Medicine* 36(3):379–387.
Panjabi, Ranee Khooshie Lal
  2010   Sacrificial Lambs of Globalization: Child Labor in the Twenty-First Century. *Journal of
          International Law and Public Policy* 37(3):421–464.
Parkinson, Constance
  1980   The Changing Pattern of Paraquat Poisoning in Man. *Histopathology* 4(2):171–183.
Pendergrast, Mark
  1999   *Uncommon Grounds: The History of Coffee and How it Transformed Our World*. New
          York: Basic Books.
Pesticide Action Network (PAN)
  2010   *Communities in Peril: Global Report on Health Impacts of Pesticide Use in Agriculture.*
          Penang, Malaysia: Pesticide Action Network Asia and the Pacific (PAN AP).
Pesticide Action Network (PAN) Pesticide Database
  2003   Human Toxicity. http://www.pesticideinfo.org/Docs/ref_toxicitytop.html, accessed
          Februrary 20, 2013.
Pfeiffer, James and Rachel Chapman
  2010   Anthropological Perspectives on Structural Adjustment and Public Health. *Annual
          Review of Anthropology* 39:149–165.
Ponte, Stefano
  2002   The 'Latte Revolution'? Regulation, Markets, and Consumption in the Global Coffee
          Chain. *World Development* 30(7):1099–1122.
Ponte, Stefano and Peter Gibbon
  2005   Quality Standards, Conventions and the Governance of Global Value Chains. *Economy
          and Society* 34(1):1–31.
Popper, Roger, Karla Andino, Mario Bustamante, Beatriz Hernandes, and Luis Rodas
  1996   Knowledge and Beliefs Regarding Agricultural Pesticides in Rural Guatemala. *Environ-
          mental Management* 20(2):241–248.
Programa de las Naciones Unidas para el Desarrollo (PNUD)
  2010   *Guatemala: Hacia un Estado para el Desarrollo*. Guatemala City, Guatemala: PNUD.
  2008   *Informe Nacional de Desarrollo Humano: Guatemala: Una Economía al Servicio del
          Desarrollo Humano?* Guatemala City, Guatemala: PNUD.
Prüss-Üstün, Annette, David Kay, Lorna Fewtrell, and Jamie Bartram
  2004   Unsafe Water, Sanitation, and Hygiene. In *Global and Regional Burden of Disease Attrib-
          utable to Selected Major Risk Factors*, Majid Essati, Alan D. Lopez, Anthony Rodgers, and
          Christopher J. L. Murray, eds. 1321–1352. Geneva: World Health Organization.
Quirós, Ronald Soto and David Díaz Arias
  2007   Mestizaje, Indígenas e Identidad Nacional en Centroamérica: De la Colonaia a las
          Repúblicas Liberales. Cuaderno de Ciencias Sociales, Costa Rica: FLACSO-Costa Rica.
Raynolds, Laura
  2002   Poverty Alleviation through Participation in Fair Trade Coffee Networks: Existing Re-
          search and Critical Issues. Background Paper, New York: The Ford Foundation.

Recio, Rogelio, Wendy A. Robbins, Guadalupe Ocampo-Gómez, Victor Borja-Aburto, Javier Morán-Martínez, John R. Froines, Rosa Ma, García Hernández, and Mariano E Cebrián
    2001   Organophosphorous Pesticide Exposure Increases the Frequency of Sperm Sex Null Aneuploidy. *Environmental Health Perspectives* 109(12):1237–1240.

Reidy, Thomas J., Rosemarie M. Bowler, Stephen S. Rauch, and George I. Pedroza
    1992   Pesticide Exposure and Neuropsychological Impairment in Migrant Farm Workers. *Archives of Clinical Neuropsychology* 7(1):85–95.

Rohlman, Diane S., Steffani R. Bailey, W. Kent Anger, and Linda McCauley
    2001   Assessment of Neurobehavioral Function with Computerized Tests in a Population of Hispanic Adolescents Working in Agriculture. *Environmental Research* 85(1):14–24.

Roldán-Tapia, Lola, Tesifón Parrón, and Fernando Sánchez-Santed
    2005   Neuropsychological Effects of Long-Term Exposure to Organophosphate Pesticides. *Neurotoxicology and Teratology* 27(2):259–266.

Ron, Aviva
    1999   NGOs in community health insurance schemes: examples from Guatemala and the Philippines. *Social Science & Medicine* 48:939–950.

Rosenstock, Linda, Matthew Keifer, William E. Daniell, Robert McConnell, and Keith Claypoole
    1991   Chronic Central Nervous System Effects of Acute Organophosphate Pesticide Intoxication. *Lancet* 338(8761):223–227.

Rudd, Rima E., Tayla Colton, and Robin Schacht
    2000   An Overview of Medical and Public Health Literature Addressing Literacy Issues: An Annotated Bibliography. Report. The National Center for the Study of Adult Learning and Literacy. Cambridge, MA: NCSALL Reports.

Rudel, Thomas K.
    2007   Changing Agents of Deforestation: From State-Initiated to Enterprise Driven Processes, 1970–2000. *Land Use Policy* 24:35–41.

Sanborn, Margaret, Donald Cole, Kathleen Kerr, and Cathy Vakil
    2004   Pesticides Literature Review. Project Report. Toronto: The Ontario College of Family Physicians.

Savitz, D. A., T. Arbuckle, D. Kaczor, and K. M. Curtis
    1997   Male Pesticide Exposure and Pregnancy Outcome. *American Journal of Epidemiology* 146:1025–1036.

Scott, James C.
    1976   *The Moral Economy of the Peasant: Rebellion and Subsistence in Southeast Asia.* New Haven, CT: Yale University Press.
    1998   *Seeing Like a State: How Certain Schemes to Improve the Human Condition Have Failed.* New Haven, CT: Yale University Press.

Seidler, A., W. Hellenbrand, B. P. Robra, P. Vieregge, P. Nischan, J. Joerg, W. H. Oertel, G. Ulm, and E. Schneider
    1996   Possible Environmental, Occupational, and Other Etiologic Factors for Parkinson's Disease: A Case-Control Study in Germany. *Neurology* 46:1275–1284.

Smit, Lidwien A. M., Berna N. van-Wendel-de-Joode, Dick Heederik, Roshini J. Peiris-John, and Wim van der Hoek
    2003   Neurological Symptoms among Sri Lankan Farmers Occupationally Exposed to Acetylcholinesterase-Inhibiting Insecticides. *American Journal of Industrial Medicine* 44(3):254–264.

Smith, Carl, Kathleen Kerr, and Ava Sadripour Esq.
    2008   Pesticide Exposure from U.S. Ports, 2001–2003. *International Journal of Occupational and Environmental Health* 14(3):176–186.

Smith, Carol, ed.
    1990   *Guatemalan Indians and the State, 1540 to 1988.* Austin: University of Texas Press.

Sparr, Pamela, ed.
    1994   *Mortgaging Women's Lives: Feminist Critiques of Structural Adjustment.* London: Zed Books.

Stiglitz, Joseph E.
  2002   *Globalization and its Discontents.* New York: W.W. Norton & Company, Inc.
  2004   Capital-Market Liberalization, Globalization, and the IMF. *Oxford Review of Economic Policy* 20(1):57–71.
Summers, Lawrence H., and Lant H. Pritchett
  1993   The Structural-Adjustment Debate. *The American Economic Review* 83(2):383–389.
Taylor, Peter Leigh
  2005   In the Market but Not of It: Fair Trade Coffee and Forest Stewardship Council Certification as Market-Based Social Change. *World Development* 33(1):129–147.
Thrupp, Lori Ann, with Gilles Bergeron and William F. Waters
  1995   *Bittersweet Harvests for Global Supermarkets: Challenges in Latin America's Agricultural Export Boom.* Washington, DC: World Resources Institute.
Topik, Steven
  2003   The Integration of the World Coffee Market. In *The Global Coffee Economy in Africa, Asia, and Latin America, 1500–1989.* William Gervase Clarence-Smith and Steven Topik, eds. 21–49. Cambridge, UK: Cambridge University Press.
United Nations Environment Programme (UNEP)
  2012   Rotterdam Convention on the Prior Informed Consent Procedure for Certain Hazardous Chemicals and Pesticides in International Trade. Electronic document www.pic.int, accessed February 20, 2013.
  2004   Status of Ratifications. http://chm.pops.int/Countries/StatusofRatifications/tabid/252/Default.aspx, accessed February 20, 2013.
  n.d.   Global Alliance for Alternatives to DDT. http://chm.pops.int/Implementation/DDT/GlobalAlliance/tabid/621/mctl/ViewDetails/EventModID/1421/EventID/136/xmid/6821/Default.aspx, accessed February 20, 2013.
University of Hawaii at Manoa
  n.d.   Coffee Berry Borer (*Hypothenemus hampei*). http://www.ctahr.hawaii.edu/site/CBBManage.aspx, accessed July 14, 2013.
Van Dijk, J. B., D. H. M. van Doesburg, A. M. A. Heijbroek, M. R. I. A. Wazir, and G. S. M. de Wolff
  1998   *The World Coffee Market.* Utrecht: Rabobank International.
Wallerstein, Nina B. and Bonnie Duran
  2006   Using Community-Based Participatory Research to Address Health Disparities. *Health Promotion Practice* 7:312.
Weller, Susan C., Trenton R. Ruebush II, and Robert E. Klein
  1997   Predicting Treatment-Seeking Behavior in Guatemala: A Comparison of the Health Services, Research and Decision-Theoretic Approaches. *Medical Anthropology Quarterly* 11(2):224–245.
Wesseling, Catharina, Matthew Keifer, Anders Ahlbom, Rob McConnell, Jai-Dong Moon, Linda Rosenstock, and Christer Hogstedt
  2002   Long-Term Neurobehavioral Effects of Mild Poisonings with Organophosphate and n-Methyl Carbamate Pesticides among Banana Workers. International *Journal of Occupational and Environmental Health* 8(1):27–34.
World Bank
  n.d. a   External debt stocks, total (DOD, current US$) http://data.worldbank.org/indicator/DT.DOD.DECT.CD, accessed February 24, 2013.
  n.d. b   Guatemala. http://data.worldbank.org/country/guatemala, accessed February 24, 2013.
World Health Organization
  2004   The Impact of Pesticides on Health. Electronic document http://www.who.int/mental_health/prevention/suicide/en/PesticidesHealth2.pdf, accessed February 20, 2013.
World Health Organization (WHO) and United Nations Environment Programme (UNEP)
  1990   *Public Health Impact of Pesticides Used in Agriculture.* Geneva, Switzerland: WHO.

Index